"PARTNERS IN PARENTING"

LETHBRIDGE & DISTRICT

Supported by:

Kiwanis Club of Green Acres

You and Your Baby

You and Your Baby

Douglas & McIntyre
Vancouver/Toronto

*in cooperation with the Health
Services and Promotion Branch,
Health and Welfare Canada and
the Canada Communication
Group—Publishing, Supply and
Services Canada*

Written by Kate Nonesuch
Catalogue number: H53-2/1991E
          94 95   2 3

Copublished by Douglas & McIntyre Ltd. in cooperation
with Health and Welfare Canada and the Canada
Communication Group—Publishing, Supply and Services
Canada

Douglas & McIntyre Ltd.
1615 Venables Street
Vancouver, British Columbia V5L 2H1

Canadian Cataloguing in Publication Data
Main entry under title:
You and your baby

  First-4th eds. published as: The Canadian mother and child.
  Includes index.
  ISBN 0-88894-713-5

  1. Pregnancy. 2. Childbirth. 3. Infants—Care.
I. Canada. Health Services and Promotion Branch. II. Title:
The Canadian mother and child.
RG525.C35 1991   618.2   C91-091650-0

Cover design by Robert MacDonald/MediaClones
Printed and bound in Canada by D. W. Friesen & Sons Ltd.
Printed on acid-free paper ∞

Contents

Preface 1
How To Use This Book 3

Chapter 1
Before You're Pregnant 4
  What kind of a parent will I be? 5
  Getting ready to have a baby 6
  It helps if you're healthy 7
  Before you get pregnant 8
  Family health 9
  Dental work 9
  Immunization 9
  Sexually transmitted diseases (STDs) 10
  Just for partners 10

Chapter 2
Human Reproduction 13
  The female organs of reproduction 13
  The male organs of reproduction 14
  How does it work? 15
  Multiple births 16
  How long does it take from start to finish? . . 17
  How fast does the baby grow? 17
  When to expect your baby 19
  How the baby grows 21

Chapter 3
Taking Care of Your Health 24
  How do I know I'm pregnant? 24

See your doctor 24
How does it feel to be pregnant? 26
   Sometimes I just feel like yelling
     and crying! 26
   I'm so tired 27
   I feel sick 27
   I get heartburn 27
   I'm constipated 28
   I get cramps in my legs 28
   What about varicose veins? 28
   My skin is all blotchy 29
   I'm getting stretch marks 29
   Hemorrhoids 29
   My underwear is always damp 30
   Danger signs 30
Keeping in touch with your doctor 31
Superstitions 31
Some special needs 32
   The young mother 32
   The older mother 33
   What does Rh factor mean? 33
Special tests 35
What about circumcision? 35
Childbirth education classes 36
Just for partners 37

Chapter 4
Eating Well 39
   What do I need to know to eat well? 39
   Healthy eating 39
      1. Milk and milk products 40
      2. Breads, cereals, pasta and rice 41

   3. Vegetables, fruits, legumes,
      nuts and seeds 41
   4. Meat, poultry, fish and eggs 42
   Extras 43
How much weight should I gain? 44
How much can I eat? 44
When should I eat? 45
What should I drink? 45
Do I need extra vitamins? 45
Can food additives and preservatives
  harm the baby? 46
Does it cost a lot to eat right? 46
I am a vegetarian. What should I eat? 47
What about alcohol? 47
Just for partners 47

Chapter 5
Daily Life while You're Pregnant 48
Sleep 48
Work 48
Parental leave 50
Daily physical activity 51
Social life 51
Smoking 52
Travel 52
Sex 53
Baths 53
Saunas and hot tubs 54
Clothes 54
Douches 54
Drugs and medication 54
Stress 55

Around the house 56
Just for partners 56

Chapter 6
How To Stay Comfortable **58**
Stand straight, sit straight 58
Making your muscles stronger 60
Tighten your pelvic muscles 61
Tighten your abdominal muscles 62
Relaxing 62
Breathe your worries away 63
Relax your whole body 63
Lying on your back 64
Lying on your side 65
Just for partners 66

Chapter 7
Getting Ready for Your Baby **67**
What does a baby need? 67
Crib 68
Clothing 69
Diapers 70
What else does the baby need? 72
Car seat 73
Getting ready to go to the hospital 73
Feeding your baby 74
Just for partners 75

Chapter 8
Having Your Baby **76**
How can I tell it's getting close? 76
Signs of labour 77

At the hospital 78
Labour and delivery 78
   How to breathe during labour
     and delivery 78
   Other ways to relax and control pain 79
   First stage 80
   Second stage 81
   Baby is here 83
   Third stage 83
Looking after the baby 84
Drugs during labour and delivery 84
Forceps and suction 86
Caesarean birth 86
Induced labour 87
Just for partners 88

Chapter 9
After Your Baby Is Born 90
   Looking after the mother 91
   How long will I stay in the hospital? 91
   More body changes 92
   How long will I need to wear a pad? 93
   When will I get my period again? 93
   My feelings are all mixed up 93
     I cry for no reason! 94
     I can't believe it really happened! 94
     I believe it! I believe it! 95
     I can handle this! 95
   Looking after your baby 96
   Rooming in or combined care 97
   Some babies need special care 97
   My baby is in an incubator 98

Getting ready to go home 98
    Help at home 98
    Fill out those forms! 99
    Birth control 99
    Part of the family 99
Just for partners 100

Chapter 10
Planning Your Family 103
Birth control pill 104
I.U.D. (intrauterine device) 104
Vaginal diaphragm with spermicidal
    jelly or cream 105
Vaginal spermicidal jelly,
    cream or foam 106
Vaginal sponge 106
Fertility awareness and natural
    family planning 106
Cervical cap 107
Condoms 107
Withdrawal 108
Sterilization 108

Chapter 11
Getting Back in Shape 109
Pelvic tilt exercise 109
    Sitting 110
    Standing 110
Pelvic floor contraction exercise (Kegel) . . . 111
Exercises for abdominal muscles 111

Chapter 12
First Days at Home **114**

Baby's head 115
Baby's face 115
Baby's legs 115
Baby's skin 116
Some early changes 116
Baby learns to trust 117
Sleeping 117
Crying 117
Looking after the cord 118
Bathing 119
  Keep the baby safe in the bath 120
  Getting ready for the bath 120
Sponge bath 121
Tub bath 123
Clothing 125
Just for partners 125

Chapter 13
Feeding Your Baby **127**

Why breast-feed? 127
Bottle-feeding 127
Breast-feeding your baby 128
  How should I hold the baby? 128
  How often should I breast-feed? 130
  I get cramps when the baby is nursing . . 130
  Is my baby getting enough milk? 130
  Keeping it up 131
  Bowel movements 132
  Can I keep breast-feeding after I go
    back to work? 132

Can I freeze my breast milk? 133
How to use frozen breast milk 134
Can I breast-feed my twins? 135
My baby came early. Can I breast-feed? 135
How long should I nurse my baby? 135
Support groups 136
Bottle-feeding your baby 136
Infant formula 136
Making the formula 137
Warming the bottle 139
Feeding the baby 139
What about burping? 141
Teaching your baby to use a cup 141
Does my baby need water? 142
Do I have to boil the water for the baby? 142
What kind of water should I use? 142
When to introduce cow's milk 143
Giving your baby solid foods 143
What should I give him first? 144
What should the texture of solid
foods be? 145
Dangerous foods 146
Adding a new food 146
Solid foods: commercial or homemade? . 147
How do I make my own baby food? . . . 147
Feeding a vegetarian baby 148
Vitamins and minerals 149
Flouride 149
Making mealtimes easy 150

Chapter 14
Your Baby's First Year

Your Baby's First Year 152
The visiting nurse 152
Growing bigger 152
Clothing 154
    Clothes for outside 154
    Clothes for inside 154
Sleeping 154
Play time 156
Exercise 157
Toys 157
Soothers 157
Sucking the thumb 158
Dental health 159
    Nursing bottle syndrome 159
    Dental problems 159
    Teething 160
Immunization 161
Travelling 163
    By car 163
    By plane 163
Just for partners 164

Chapter 15
Your Baby Grows

Your Baby Grows 165
First month 166
Second month 168
Third and fourth months 168
Fifth and sixth months 169
Seventh and eighth months 170
Ninth and tenth months 170
Eleventh to fourteenth months 171

Does my child have a problem? 171
How can I help my baby learn? 172
Play 172
Discipline 173
Setting rules 174
Sometimes I get so mad! 174
What should I do if I
    think I might hurt my child? 175
Make time for your baby 175
Fears 176
Older children 176
Grandparents and other relatives 177
Sitters 177
Day care while you work 178
    How will my child adjust to
        going to day care? 179
    What kind of day care is available? 180
    How do I choose? 180
    Contracts 181
    Subsidies 181
Just for partners 182

Chapter 16
Safety and First Aid 184
Don't let injuries happen! 184
When do injuries happen? 185
Why do injuries happen? 185
Be prepared 186
What kinds of injuries are most
    common for kids? 187
How do I keep my child safe in the car? . . . 187
    Choose the right seat for your child 188

General car safety 189
Safe furniture for children 190
    Playpen 190
    Crib 190
    Baby seat 190
    Highchair 191
    Walkers 191
Making your home safe 192
    Kitchen 192
    Bathroom 192
    Living room 193
    Bedroom 193
    Halls and stairs 194
    Basement and storage rooms 194
Pets 195
Other things to remember 195
Outdoor safety 196
Boating safety 197
Farm safety 197
Snowmobile safety 197
When to call for help 198
Burns 199
Poisons 200
Choking (baby) 200
Choking (child) 203
Rescue breathing 205
    For a baby 205
    For a child 206
When a child is unconscious 207
Falls, sprains and fractures 209
Lumps and bumps on the head 210
Cuts and bleeding 211

    Small cuts 211
    Heavy bleeding 211
  Bites and stings 212
    Animal or human bites 212
    Bee and insect stings 212
  Slivers 213
  Something in the eye 213
  Objects in the ears 213
  Objects in the nose 214
  Frostbite 214
  Sunburn 215
  Sunstroke and heat exhaustion 215

Chapter 17
When Your Baby Is Sick 216
  Crying 216
  How can I tell if he is sick? 216
  Can my sick child go to day care? 217
  What should I tell the doctor? 218
  How to take a baby's temperature 218
  What should I do when
    my baby has a fever? 219
  Convulsions 219
  Stomach aches 220
  Diarrhea 221
  How should I feed the baby after
    he is better? 222
  Throwing up 223
  Constipation 224
  Hiccups 224
  Colic 225
    What can I do? 225

Skin troubles 227
    Diaper rash 227
    Prickly heat 228
    Eczema 228
    Impetigo 229
Thrush 230
Colds 231
Sore throat 232
Croup 232
Earache 233
Parasites 234
    Lice 234
    Scabies 234
    Pinworms 235

Appendix 1
Emergency Delivery 236

Keep the mother and baby clean 236
Labour and delivery 237
Taking care of the baby 238
After the baby is born 239
Looking after the mother 240
Emergencies that sometimes happen 241
    The baby is already born
      when you get there 241
    The baby is born bottom first 241
    The baby is born on
      the way to the hospital 242

Index 244

Preface

For the past fifty years, the Department of National Health and Welfare has provided Canadians with information on mother and child care. Its first major book, *The Canadian Mother's Book*, came out in 1921. *The Canadian Mother and Child* appeared in 1940 and was reproduced yearly with small changes; it had a major revision in 1953 and was rewritten in 1967 and 1979. It has been used by parents, teachers, health-care professionals and students.

This new edition is up to date, accurate and easy to read. It provides practical information in an informal format. Questions and answers are used to make it easy to find particular details as the reader needs them.

The book deals with family life in the larger community. Most Canadian children are born into a family and cared for by their parents. Of course, there are many differences in cultures, families and individual lifestyles. However, a wide network of community support and services is available to every family. One of the important roles of this book is to make the reader aware of this network.

The new title reflects the way parents today are sharing responsibility for looking after children. *You and Your Baby* is aimed at both mothers and fathers. Today, many fathers are taking a bigger share of day-to-day child care, and many mothers have careers that are a major focus of their lives. More children are spending time at day-care centres or in the care of someone who is neither mother nor father.

You and Your Baby reflects another change in thinking as well. More and more people are taking responsibility for their own good health by good eating, exercise and a healthy lifestyle; these things help to prevent illness and injuries. The book stresses healthy living and good communication with health care professionals, and encourages parents to be part of the health care team in their community.

It has been suggested that the book be divided into two books, one on pregnancy and delivery and another on infant care. However, the single volume has been kept so readers can see how a healthy way of life during pregnancy leads naturally to a healthy way of life for the whole family.

We hope that new mothers and fathers will find practical help in planning and caring for their children. We also hope that the book will give them confidence in their ability to be effective parents.

The Department is most grateful to the many people and groups who helped prepare this revised edition, with special thanks to writer Kate Nonesuch and illustrator Suzanne Labelle. Their professional expertise and knowledge have helped make a book that will continue to help Canadian families in years to come.

How To Use This Book

Probably you will not sit down and read this book all at once.

You may want to go back to it often and read some parts over again when you need them. The first chapter is about preparing for pregnancy, and the second talks about becoming pregnant. Chapters 4, 5, 6 and 7 will answer many of your questions about pregnancy and preparing for the baby. Chapters 8 and 9 are about delivery and the stay in the hospital. The rest of the book deals with looking after your baby.

Use the Table of Contents at the beginning of the book to find the chapter you want.

Sometimes you may want to find something quickly, without reading a whole chapter. For example, you may have heartburn and want to know what to do. The index in the back of the book will help. Look up "heartburn," and you will find all the pages that mention heartburn. Turn to those pages, and look for the word "heartburn." Read what you need.

The term "doctor" is used all through this book, but the person who can help you may also be a nurse, nutritionist or other care provider.

In "Just for Partners," a special section at the end of most chapters, partners and fathers will find some help with their role in pregnancy, delivery and parenting.

Chapter 1

Before You're Pregnant

Do I want a baby now?

Can we afford it?

Is there room in my home and my life for a new child?

If you are thinking about having a baby, you will probably be thinking about these questions.

Many other questions may be running through your mind, too:

- Who comes first, parent or child?
- What if we can't agree on how to raise the baby?
- What does a baby need?
- How will being a parent affect my work?
- How will a baby affect my sex life?
- What will the other children think? How can I help them accept a new baby?

This book will answer many of your questions, but not all of them. Your own preferences, beliefs and lifestyle will shape your decisions about having a baby.

When two people raise a baby, each person has ideas about how to be a parent. Often the two people have different ideas, especially about discipline. If you and your partner talk things over before you get pregnant, there won't be as

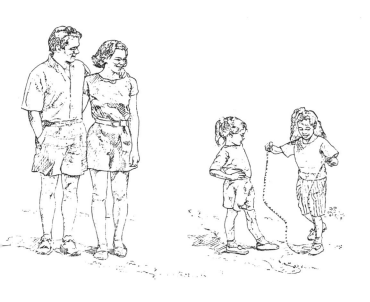

many surprises after the baby comes; you will be well prepared to work together to create a strong family.

If you are a single parent, working out your ideas about raising a child will help keep things clear. What do you need to make your relationship with your child work well? Talk to someone you trust, perhaps another single parent, or your parents, or a friend.

What kind of a parent will I be?
Look around you. Think of all the parents you know—your parents, your aunt and uncle, your

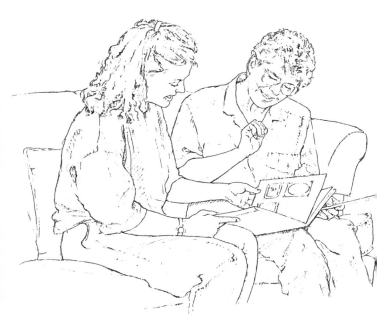

friends or neighbours. Parents are always learning—by watching and talking to other parents,
by going to classes, or by reading books on better
parenting. You don't know any perfect parents,
because nobody does everything right all the
time. You won't be a perfect parent, either. Trust
yourself to figure things out and to find out what
you need to know. Trust yourself, and your baby
will trust you too.

Getting ready to have a baby
Having a baby can be wonderful. It may make
you feel part of a chain that joins you to your

parents, grandparents and great-grandparents.

There is nothing more interesting than a new baby who has lots to learn about the world and about his new family. A new person is coming to life, and you are in on it from the start. What kind of a person will this new baby grow up to be? To a great extent, it depends on you.

However, no matter how exciting they are, babies do not solve other problems. If you are having trouble at work or with your partner, try to work things out before you have the baby. If you don't feel well or are always tired, see your doctor. Start to eat better and exercise more. Getting your life in order will make it easier to look after a baby; you will have more time and energy to enjoy being a parent.

It helps if you're healthy

You need to eat well and to get enough exercise and sleep.

Good eating will help you avoid many problems, and a healthy mother will quickly get her strength and her energy back after the baby is born.

Cigarettes, drugs and alcohol can harm the baby. You may hear other people say, "Oh, I drank when I was pregnant and the baby was fine. My doctor said it was okay." However, things have changed. Some new studies show that even a small amount of alcohol can have serious effects on your baby. If you smoke or drink, your baby is more likely to be born early or to be small. A baby who is born more than six weeks early, or who weighs less than 2.5 kg (5.5 lb.), is more likely to be weak or to have physical or mental problems.

Before you get pregnant

If you want to be pregnant, or if you are having sex and not using birth control, talk to your doctor now about pregnancy.

Your doctor will give you a checkup and ask you about your health and your family's health. You may be asked to have some tests—hemoglobin tests to check for nutritional anemia, a urinalysis, Rh typing, tests for sexually transmitted diseases, also called STDs, and a Pap smear.

The doctor will ask you lots of questions:

- Do you have regular periods?
- Have you been pregnant before?
- Have you had a miscarriage or an abortion?
- What drugs are you using?
- How much alcohol do you drink?
- Do you smoke?
- What is your normal weight?
- What are your usual eating habits?
- Do you have allergies?
- Is your immunization up to date?
- What illnesses have you had? Have you had German measles?
- Have you been taking birth control pills? If so, the doctor may suggest you wait a few months after you stop taking the pill before

you get pregnant. You will need to use some other kind of birth control while you are waiting. See Chapter 10, "Planning Your Family," for more information.

The first few weeks of pregnancy are very important for the baby, but this is a time when you do not know for sure if you are pregnant. If it is possible that you are, there are some tests, treatments and medicines you shouldn't have. Tell any doctor you see that you might be pregnant.

Family health
Your doctor will take a complete health history. He or she will want to know about illnesses in your background. Are there any diseases that run in your family?

Are you related to someone who had a child with birth defects? Tell your doctor, even if it is not a close relation. Are you distantly related to the father of your child? If so, you may need to have some genetic tests done.

Dental work
Go to the dentist for a checkup. The dentist should do any needed work before you are pregnant.

Immunization
Are you planning to travel? If you will need a vaccination, do it now, because it may be dangerous to have it done while you are pregnant.

Have you had German measles? German measles early in a pregnancy can cause problems with the baby's ears, eyes, nervous system or heart. If you had German measles as a child, you will be immune now. You can be tested to find out if you are immune to German measles.

If you are not immune, you can be immunized against it. You should not get pregnant for at least three months after this immunization.

Sexually transmitted diseases (STDs)

STDs are diseases like AIDS, chlamydia, syphilis, gonorrhea and herpes. They are diseases you can catch while having sex. If you have had many different sex partners, or if your partner has had many different partners, you are at risk of catching an STD. If you are an injection drug user, you can get some STDs from sharing needles or syringes.

If you have an STD, you could give it to your baby, either before or during birth. Talk to your doctor about STDs.

Just for partners

This is a happy and exciting time for new fathers. If you are the father of the baby, or if you are the friend or partner of someone who is pregnant, there are many things you can do to get involved.

New parents will want to think about the differences a baby will make. Share your feelings with your partner. Are you ready to make some changes in your life to look after a baby? Do you need to change your work schedule so you can be around more? Can you get up at night to look after the baby? Talk to your friends who have babies. Ask them about the difference a baby makes. They can tell you how wonderful babies are, and how they fill up your days and nights.

You and your partner may want to go to the doctor together, since you both will have questions to ask. If you are the father, talk to the doctor about your health and your family background.

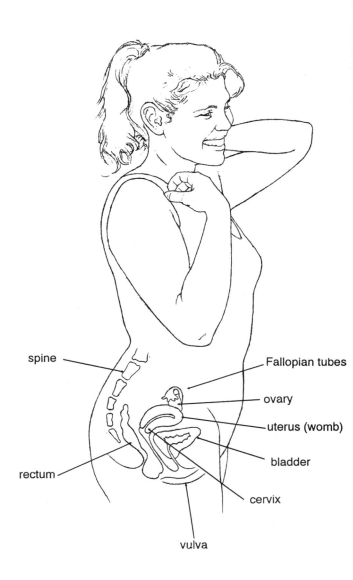

spine

Fallopian tubes

ovary

uterus (womb)

bladder

rectum

cervix

vulva

Chapter 2

Human Reproduction

When a woman is pregnant, her body changes so she can take care of her baby before and after birth.

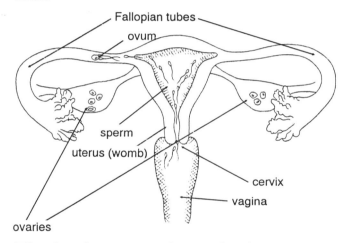

Fallopian tubes

ovum

sperm

uterus (womb)

cervix

vagina

ovaries

The female organs of reproduction

The uterus lies between the bladder and other organs in the large intestine. Before pregnancy it is only about 8 cm (3 in.) long, but by the end of the pregnancy it fills up most of the space in the abdomen.

Near the top of the uterus, the Fallopian tubes extend out towards the ovaries. The tubes are 7 to

10 cm (3 to 4 in.) long. Each tube has a fringed end, and the fringes can move freely. The ovaries are found at the end of the tubes. The ovaries make the eggs, or ova. One egg is called an ovum; when there is more than one, they are called ova.

At the lower end of the uterus, there is an opening from the uterus into the vagina. This neck of the uterus is called the cervix.

All of these organs are in the pelvis; the pelvis is the name for the hipbones and the muscles and tissues that make up the pelvic floor. These muscles are intertwined to form a hammock that supports the organs of the abdomen and pelvis.

The male organs of reproduction

The main sex organs of the male are the penis and the testicles. The testicles hang between the legs in a pouch called the scrotum. The testicles make

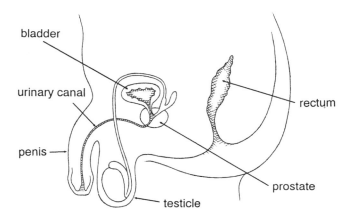

a white liquid called semen, which contains sperm cells. A sperm is much smaller than an ovum.

During sexual intercourse, semen will spurt from the penis into the vagina. The sperm start to swim up the vagina to meet an egg cell or ovum.

How does it work?

Every month or so, one of the woman's ovaries releases an ovum. The ovum moves into the large end of the Fallopian tube and along the tube to the uterus. It takes three or four days to reach the uterus.

When a woman and a man have sexual intercourse, the sperm move up the vagina, into the uterus and along the Fallopian tubes, searching for an ovum.

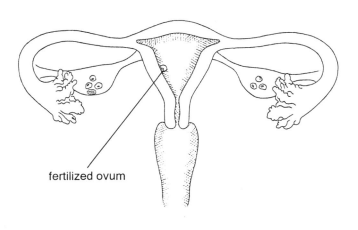

fertilized ovum

If the couple is not using birth control, and if the ovary has released an ovum, one sperm will get to the ovum before any other sperm does. The first sperm to reach the ovum enters it. This is called fertilization. No other sperm can get into the ovum after this. The fertilized ovum can develop into a baby.

The sperm from the father and the ovum from the mother each provide the new baby with some features. She might have her father's eyes and her mother's nose, or vice versa.

Multiple births

Most of the time, the ovaries let go of only one ovum, and one fetus develops.

Sometimes two ova leave the ovaries at the same time. Two sperm cells join the two ova, and two fetuses develop. These twins are called fraternal twins. They are not exactly the same but are just like any two children born to the same parents. They may be the same sex, or they may be a brother and a sister. Once in a while, more ova are released, and three, four or more babies develop.

Sometimes two babies are made from one ovum and one sperm. After the sperm has fertilized the ovum, the ovum splits into two parts. Twins again! But this time they are identical twins. They are exactly the same, either two boys or two girls.

How long does it take from start to finish?

The baby will be born about nine months later, or about 266 days after fertilization. That is about 280 days after the beginning of your last period.

The chart will help you figure out when to expect your baby. The light type is the first day of your last period, and the bold type under it is your due date. For example, if your last period started on January 25, your due date is November 1.

How fast does the baby grow?

A fertilized ovum is called an embryo. The embryo moves along the Fallopian tube, growing as it moves. The picture shows how it gets bigger. It grows by dividing. First it divides itself into two cells. Then each of those parts divides in half, so there are four. Each of those divides to make eight, and so on.

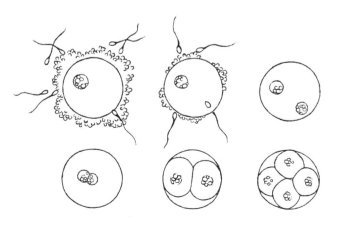

In a few days, the embryo moves into the uterus. It attaches itself to the lining of the uterus, which has been prepared to nourish the embryo. The embryo keeps getting bigger and starts to grow special cells that will become the brain, stomach and other organs of the body.

Then the embryo grows very quickly. At twelve weeks it is called a fetus, and it continues to grow rapidly. It grows inside a bag of fluid called the amniotic sac. The amniotic sac keeps the baby safe. Part of the outside of the sac is very close to the side of the uterus. This part is called the afterbirth, or the placenta. The placenta is full of blood vessels that take nourishment and oxygen from the mother's blood and pass it on to the baby. The placenta takes waste products from the baby's blood and passes them back to the mother's blood so the mother's body can get rid of them. Infections, alcohol and drugs (nicotine and others) can be passed through the placenta to the baby. Everything moves back and forth through the placenta, but the mother's own blood does not flow through the baby.

A long cord stretches from the placenta to the baby. It is called the umbilical cord. The baby's blood flows through the cord to the placenta and back again.

When to expect your baby

The top line of each pair shows the day of the month; the bold line below shows the day your baby is expected. Each row is also labelled on both sides of the chart by the conception month and the two possible months of arrival.

Conception month	1	2	3	4	5	6	7	8	9	10	11	12	13	14	15	16	17	18	19	20	21	22	23	24	25	26	27	28	29	30	31	Expected
January	8	9	10	11	12	13	14	15	16	17	18	19	20	21	22	23	24	25	26	27	28	29	30	31	1	2	3	4	5	6	7	October / November
February	8	9	10	11	12	13	14	15	16	17	18	19	20	21	22	23	24	25	26	27	28	29	30	1	2	3	4	5	6			November / December
March	8	9	10	11	12	13	14	15	16	17	18	19	20	21	22	23	24	25	26	27	28	29	30	31	1	2	3	4	5	6	7	December / January
April	8	9	10	11	12	13	14	15	16	17	18	19	20	21	22	23	24	25	26	27	28	29	30	31	1	2	3	4	5	6		January / February
May	8	9	10	11	12	13	14	15	16	17	18	19	20	21	22	23	24	25	26	27	28	1	2	3	4	5	6	7	8	9	10	February / March
June	8	9	10	11	12	13	14	15	16	17	18	19	20	21	22	23	24	25	26	27	28	29	30	31	1	2	3	4	5	6		March / April
July	8	9	10	11	12	13	14	15	16	17	18	19	20	21	22	23	24	25	26	27	28	29	30	1	2	3	4	5	6	7	8	April / May
August	8	9	10	11	12	13	14	15	16	17	18	19	20	21	22	23	24	25	26	27	28	29	30	31	1	2	3	4	5	6	7	May / June
September	8	9	10	11	12	13	14	15	16	17	18	19	20	21	22	23	24	25	26	27	28	29	30	1	2	3	4	5	6	7		June / July
October	8	9	10	11	12	13	14	15	16	17	18	19	20	21	22	23	24	25	26	27	28	29	30	31	1	2	3	4	5	6	7	July / August
November	8	9	10	11	12	13	14	15	16	17	18	19	20	21	22	23	24	25	26	27	28	29	30	31	1	2	3	4	5	6		August / September
December	8	9	10	11	12	13	14	15	16	17	18	19	20	21	22	23	24	25	26	27	28	29	30	1	2	3	4	5	6	7	8	September / October

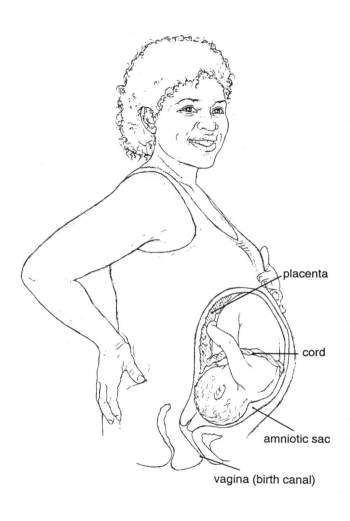

placenta

cord

amniotic sac

vagina (birth canal)

How the baby grows

Weeks after your last period	How long is the fetus?	How much does it weigh?	What's happening?
4	0.2 mm (1/100 in.)	almost nothing	The embryo digs into the lining of the uterus.
6	1 cm (0.4 in.)	almost nothing	Its head is very big compared to the rest of the body. It has a little tail, which disappears later. The brain is growing. The heart and stomach and intestines start to form.
8	2.5 cm (1 in.)	1 g (1/30 oz.)	The face looks like a person's. Eyes are shut. Legs, arms, fingers and toes are forming.
12	7.5 cm (3 in.)	30 g (1 oz.)	Sex organs are formed. The kidneys start to make urine. It is now called a fetus.
16	16 cm (6.5 in.)	120 g (4 oz.)	Soft hair covers the body. The mother may feel the fetus move. Fingernails and toenails are forming.

Weeks after your last period	How long is the fetus?	How much does it weigh?	What's happening?
20	25.4 cm (10 in.)	397 g (14 oz.)	The heartbeat can be heard through a stethoscope. The fetus sucks its thumb and hiccups. Hair, eyelashes and eyebrows are all in place.
24	30.4 cm (12 in.)	680 g (1.5 lb.)	The skin is wrinkled. The eyes are open.
28	35 cm (14 in.)	1134 g (2.5 lb.)	The fetus gains more body fat. It is more active and practises breathing.
34	44.5 cm (17.5 in.)	1814 g (4 lb.)	The fetus responds to sounds. It sleeps and wakes up. It may move into the birth position. It is gaining immunities from its mother.
40	50 cm (20 in.)	3175–3402 g (7–7.5 lb.)	It is now ready to be born. The skin is covered with vernix, a creamy material that protects it. Lungs are fully formed.

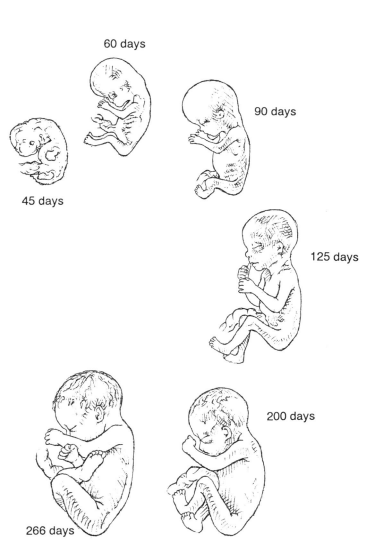

60 days

90 days

45 days

125 days

200 days

266 days

23

Chapter 3

Taking Care of Your Health

How do I know I'm pregnant?

- You miss your period.
- You have to urinate more often.
- Your breasts are full and tingling. You may be able to see the veins under the skin, because more blood is flowing to the breasts to help get them ready for nursing. Small bumps around the nipple may stick out, and the nipples may get darker.
- You may feel sick. Some women do, especially in the morning. You may vomit occasionally, or not feel like eating; however, you probably won't feel sick after the third month.

See your doctor

Call your doctor as soon as you think you might be pregnant. When your period is two weeks late, your doctor can arrange for you to have a urine test to see if you are pregnant. Sometimes people use a pregnancy test from the drugstore. These tests are not always accurate.

If you have had a pre-pregnancy checkup, your doctor will have taken a complete history. If not, or if you have a new doctor, here are some of the things you will be asked:

- Are your periods regular?
- Have you ever been pregnant before?
- Is your immunization up to date?
- What medical problems do you have?
- How much alcohol do you drink?
- Do you smoke?
- Do you use drugs?
- What medicine do you take?
- Do you sleep well?
- Do you work shifts?
- What is your diet like?
- What is your usual weight?
- What illnesses are there in your family?
- Do you work or live somewhere where the air or water is not safe, or where there are other dangers?
- Have you been around anyone with German measles or other illnesses?

Your doctor will also check your weight, blood pressure and reflexes; your eyes, ears, nose, throat, teeth and gums; your heart, lungs and kidneys; and your breasts, abdomen, ankles and feet. You will be given an internal exam to check your vagina, cervix and uterus. You will also need to have some urine and blood tests done.

The doctor will check the size of your uterus, and the size and shape of your pelvis, so that he or she can keep track of changes during your pregnancy and plan ahead to deliver your baby.

Ask the doctor to tell you what the tests say. The more you know, the more confident you'll feel, so ask about anything you don't understand.

You should visit your dentist to make sure your mouth is healthy and there are no infections. Be sure to tell your dentist you are pregnant. You can continue to have regular dental care, but if you need special treatment, your dentist will check with your doctor to make sure the procedure is safe for you and your baby.

If you see any other doctors, tell them you are pregnant so they won't give you dangerous tests or X-rays.

How does it feel to be pregnant?

Pregnancy is an emotional time for both partners. You will probably feel a mixture of excitement, joy, fear and anger. There are many changes in your body, and sometimes these changes will bother you. Fortunately, all these problems don't happen to everyone, and they don't occur all at the same time. Here are some suggestions for making yourself more comfortable while you are pregnant. Choose the symptom that fits you and ignore the rest.

Sometimes I just feel like yelling and crying!

You may feel "up" and "down" a lot more when you are pregnant. You may feel sad or worried, or you might cry or get angry about little things. You may laugh one minute and cry the next. Mood changes are normal when you are pregnant.

If you feel too far down, or if you can't shake a bad mood, tell your doctor. Moods are caused by hormone changes.

Be sure to tell your family and friends how you are feeling. If they understand how you feel, they may be able to help cheer you up. In any case, just getting your feelings out may make you feel better.

I'm so tired

There is a special tired feeling in the first two or three months of pregnancy. Suddenly you feel so tired you can hardly move—you may even fall asleep when someone is talking to you. The best thing to do is to get lots of sleep, at least eight hours at night, and a nap in the afternoon if possible.

I feel sick

Feeling sick may be one of the first signs of pregnancy. You may feel sick any time, but often it happens when you get up in the morning. Try some of these tips to make you feel better:

- Eat a few dry crackers before you get up.
- Get out of bed slowly.
- Eat four or five small meals a day, not three big ones.
- Cut down on greasy foods.

I get heartburn

If your throat or stomach start to burn about an hour after a meal, it may be heartburn. Some people find a glass of milk helps, or some other bland food like pudding, yogurt or a banana. Eating several small meals instead of a couple of big ones may make you feel better. Eat slowly, and avoid fatty foods or ones that cause gas. Ask your doctor about a safe antacid.

I'm constipated

Women often get constipated when they are pregnant. Foods with lots of fibre or bulk, like whole-wheat bread, bran cereals, dried fruit, and fresh fruits and vegetables will help prevent constipation. Drink lots of water to keep yourself regular.

It may help to take a walk every day. Don't take a laxative unless your doctor prescribes it.

I get cramps in my legs

Cramps come more often near the end of the pregnancy, mostly at night. Stretch the leg or foot. **Do not rub it**. If you have cramps in the calf of your leg, stretch your leg out. You can also lie down and get someone to press on your knee while bending your foot up toward the knee, or put some weight on your knee while you bend your foot up. A warm bath often helps.

What about varicose veins?

Near the end of pregnancy, the baby presses on the big blood vessels going to your legs and feet. The veins in the legs swell up. The best way to stop the swelling is to lie with your feet up. When you have to stand, change your position often. Wear loose stockings and underwear to help prevent varicose veins.

If your doctor suggests you wear elastic support stockings, put them on before you get out of bed and before you put any weight on your legs. You may have to put blocks of wood under the foot of your bed to lift it up, so that you can lie with your feet higher than your head. The blocks shouldn't be higher than 15 cm (6 in.).

My skin is all blotchy

You may see dark patches on your skin. If your skin is very light-coloured, the patches may show up clearly. If your skin is darker, the patches will probably be less noticeable. These dark patches are normal and will fade. They may come up on your hands or face, or you may have a dark line from your navel down to your pubic hair.

I'm getting stretch marks

Stretch marks are dark streaks on your abdomen, breasts, thighs or buttocks. They may be indented a little, and sometimes they are itchy or sore. You get them because your skin has to stretch when you gain so much weight so quickly. When the baby is born and you lose the weight, the dark lines will start to fade, but some marks may never go away completely. Moisture cream will relieve the itchiness and the dry skin, but it doesn't make the marks disappear.

Hemorrhoids

Hemorrhoids are varicose veins in the rectal area. They may be outside or inside the rectum. They get bigger when you are pregnant, but usually they go away when the baby is born. When they hurt, try sitting in a warm bath for about twenty minutes, morning and night. An ice pack or cold cloths may help, and your doctor may recommend an ointment for them. Try not to get constipated, since constipation will put extra pressure on your hemorrhoids.

My underwear is always damp
There is always some moisture in the vagina, but during pregnancy there is more than usual, because of the hormonal changes. If your underwear is always wet, if there is a greenish stain or if your vaginal area is itchy, talk to your doctor.

Danger signs
Call your doctor at once if you have any of these symptoms:
- Fluid comes out of the vagina.
- The baby stops moving for a day. You will feel the baby start to move about the fifth month. Once it starts, you will feel it many times a day.
- Blood, even a little, comes from the vagina.
- Your ankles or feet suddenly swell. Press on the swelling for a few seconds, then take your finger off. If the skin is indented where you pressed it, call your doctor. Swelling of the feet and ankles in the evening is normal at the end of a pregnancy, but it should go away after a night's rest.

- You gain weight suddenly.
- You have a headache that does not go away.
- You can't see well—everything is blurry or you have black spots in front of your eyes.
- You have a pain in the pit of your stomach.
- You keep throwing up.
- You have chills and fever.

Keeping in touch with your doctor

Your doctor will talk to you about how often to come in for a checkup. For the first six or seven months, it may be about once a month. Later in your pregnancy, your visits will be closer together.

At each visit, the doctor or nurse will weigh you, check your blood pressure, take urine and blood samples for tests, and check on the baby's movements and position.

Between visits, keep track of how you feel so you can tell the doctor if anything changes. Your doctor will want to know how you are getting along. He or she will ask you if there are changes in the baby's movements, or if you have pain, bleeding or dizziness.

As the weeks go by, you will probably have many questions popping into your mind. Keep track of them so you can ask your doctor or nurse.

Superstitions

You will hear many stories about how to tell what the baby will be like. Some people say that if you have heartburn, your baby will have a lot of hair. You will hear that if you carry your baby in front, you will have a boy, or if you carry wide you will have a girl. Some people will say they can read your tea leaves to tell the sex of the baby. None of these stories is true.

If you are worried about something, ask; don't rely on old stories. When you have clear answers to your questions, you can stop worrying.

Some special needs

Some women find it very stressful to be pregnant. If you have special needs, you can find help in the community. If you have trouble getting enough to eat, if you don't have a place to live, if you have no emotional support or if you need protection from violence, tell someone what is going on. If you don't know where to go for help, start by calling your public health unit or the local community centre.

The young mother

If you are under eighteen, you have special needs. You are changing physically, mentally and emotionally as you move from adolescence into adulthood.

Probably you didn't plan this pregnancy. It may have disrupted your relationship with your family and friends; you may have quit school because you are pregnant. Suddenly, when you need help the most, you may find yourself nearly alone.

You can help your baby by going to a doctor as soon as you think you are pregnant. Keep going to the doctor while you are pregnant, and ask about your diet. Eating well is important for you as well as for your baby. The next chapter talks about eating well when you are pregnant.

If you have a family to support you, ask them to help you follow the doctor's instructions.

If you don't have a family to help, talk to someone you trust. Some schools have special classes for young mothers. Your public health unit is a good place to look for help; some have prenatal classes especially for teenage mothers. If you talk to other mothers your own age, you may be able to help each other cope.

The older mother

If you are over thirty-five, you have special needs. Older women have a harder time than younger women in some ways and an easier time in other ways. It is important to see your doctor as soon as you think you are pregnant. There may be slightly higher risks for the baby, so your doctor may recommend prenatal diagnosis.

Sometimes there is some confusion about whether a missed period means you are pregnant or if it is the start of menopause. Your doctor will do a pregnancy test if you think you might be pregnant.

What does Rh factor mean?

Most people (85 per cent) have something in their

blood called the Rh factor. We call them Rh positive. The rest of the people (15 per cent) don't have this Rh factor. We call them Rh negative. If you are Rh negative and the baby's father is Rh positive, the baby may be Rh positive. It is possible for some of the Rh factor from the baby's blood to pass into your blood, and then your body will try to fight off the Rh factor. If this is your first baby, the baby will probably not be affected, unless you have had a blood transfusion of Rh positive blood, or you have already had a miscarriage or an abortion of an Rh positive fetus.

If you are Rh negative and your baby is Rh positive, the doctor will keep checking your blood to see if you are reacting to your baby's blood. If you are, your baby may have anemia (not enough red blood cells) and jaundice (yellow tint of the skin). Usually this clears within a few days. Sometimes the baby may need a blood transfusion.

After your baby is born, your doctor will give you an injection of a medicine to help control the Rh factor in your next pregnancy. It makes sure that if your next baby is Rh positive, your body will not react against it. To avoid problems, Rh negative mothers will receive an injection towards the end of pregnancy and after the baby is born.

Many babies have jaundice for a few days or weeks after they are born. This is not the same as Rh disease.

Special tests

Amniocentesis: A needle is passed through the frozen abdomen, uterus and amniotic sac. Fluid is taken and sent to the lab for tests. Amniocentesis is used to reveal certain genetic disorders.

Ultrasound: Sound waves are passed through your abdomen and bounce back from the fetus, placenta and your organs onto a video screen. Ultrasound is used to check the position of the placenta and the development of the fetus, or to see if you are carrying twins, or to determine your due date.

If you have amniocentesis, which is sometimes called "amnio," the doctor will know the sex of the fetus. If you have ultrasound, you might find out its sex. There is no other way to be certain of the sex; however, these tests are never done simply to find out the sex of the fetus.

What about circumcision?

Before the baby is born, think about circumcision. Circumcision is an operation done on the penis of the baby boy to remove a piece of the foreskin. It is usually done when the baby is a few days old. You will need to sign a consent form for the operation if you want your son to be circumcised.

Most children's doctors feel there is no medical reason for boys to be routinely circumcised. Some people have their baby circumcised for religious reasons. Here are some facts to consider:

- The operation is a short one, and the baby will usually heal from it in seven to ten days.
- The baby will feel some pain.
- Complications are rare but do happen occasionally.

If you are not sure what you want to do, discuss this with your doctor.

Childbirth education classes

The best place to get good information and answers to your questions about having a baby is a prenatal class. It is also a good place to share experiences with other expectant parents. Most classes include partners, but some are for women only and others are just for teenagers.

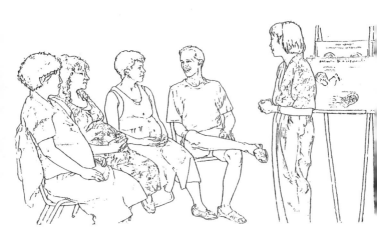

Your instructor will talk about what is happening inside your body as the baby develops. You will get lots of information on nutrition and help in figuring out what to eat; you will be able to discuss your feelings about the pregnancy and about changes in your way of living. The class usually talks about sexuality and parenting. As well, you will learn how to do some exercises that will help you get ready for the birth.

Most classes have films, discussion and room for questions. Often you will go with your class to visit the hospital. How long you will stay in the hospital varies from community to community; you will learn what your options are in your community and what help is available to you after you go home with your baby.

Talk to your doctor or your public health unit about when and where the classes are held. Childbirth education classes are good places to learn about pregnancy and childbirth. As you learn more, your worries will disappear. You will be able to make decisions about your pregnancy and feel like you are in charge. You'll have more fun.

Just for partners

What can you do? She will be making many changes in her regular patterns, getting more rest, and eating different foods in different ways. Walk through her day with her, and make some changes in your own life to match hers so you will feel like you're in this together. Try to plan a schedule that will help both of you get ready for the baby.

You will have questions about the developing baby and about your role. You might go to the doctor with her so you can share the information. Then, when things come up to bother her, you may be able to suggest a solution. Go to childbirth education classes with her. Talking to others can really give you a sense of what is usual; it helps to know that many of your feelings are natural. You can learn to be a labour coach and get ready to be there when the baby is born.

Listen to her. She will want to tell you what's going on. She may be moody and unsure of herself, and you may be feeling the same way. Sharing your thoughts and feelings with each other will help you work through this time.

Try to get on the same schedule. If she needs lots of little meals, eat lots of little meals with her. Since she needs more rest, go to bed early or do something quiet. Don't go off to a late party by yourself or expect her to come with you.

If you have been thinking about making a switch to a healthier lifestyle, why not do it together? If you want to quit smoking, drink less, eat better and get more exercise, there will never be a better time. It will help make the pregnancy easier for both of you, and after the baby is born you will have more energy to enjoy being a parent. As well, it's great for a baby to grow up in a family with a healthy lifestyle.

All of these things will add to your relationship and will make you feel involved with the baby before it is born.

Chapter 4

Eating Well

Eating well is important for you and the baby. During pregnancy you supply all the nutrients to your developing baby. If you eat well, you will likely feel good, have more energy for your daily activities and be well prepared for breast-feeding. Eating properly greatly affects the future health of your baby.

What do I need to know to eat well?

You need to know which foods to eat for good health. You need to know how to plan meals that will not cost too much, and you need to know how to store and cook foods so that they keep their nutrients.

There are many people who can help you eat well. If you go to a prenatal class, you will learn about eating well. Your doctor and your public health nurse can help, too. If you have special dietary needs because of health problems, the nurse or doctor can refer you to a public health nutritionist or a dietitian.

Do you have trouble getting to the store? Are you short of money? You can't figure out what you should eat? Ask for help.

Healthy eating

Enjoy a variety of foods every day for good

health. Choose foods each day from four major food groups:

1. milk and milk products
2. breads, cereals, pasta and rice
3. vegetables, fruits, legumes, nuts and seeds
4. meat, poultry, fish and eggs

Together, these food groups will give you and the baby the more than fifty elements that are needed for health and growth. No one food group can supply all these elements in the amount you need.

1. Milk and milk products

This group contains milk and foods made of milk like yogurt and cheese. These foods give you calcium, vitamin D and some of the B vitamins, vitamin A and protein. The calcium in milk is very important for building the baby's bones and teeth. Protein, vitamin A and vitamin D will also help make strong bones and teeth.

One per cent, two per cent or skimmed milk are just as good for you as whole milk, but you don't get as many calories.

You need more milk when you are pregnant. You should have about one litre (four cups) a day. If you don't like to drink milk, think of other ways to put it into your meals. Try a milkshake. Make soup with milk, or a sauce for vegetables. Eat it on cereals or make puddings. You can eat cheese or yogurt instead of milk.

You cannot replace what milk and milk products give you with a vitamin pill or calcium tablets. If you can't take milk and other milk products, you need to change your selection of foods or take other steps. Ask for help.

2. *Breads, cereals, pasta and rice*

Foods from this group give you carbohydrates, which are the most desirable source of energy. They are the fuel to keep you going. They are also important because they have B vitamins, iron and fibre.

Try to use whole-wheat flour, regular oatmeal and brown rice, which are not highly processed and give you more vitamins and more fibre. Some of the vitamins and iron lost in processing are replaced in enriched products such as pasta. Check the list of ingredients on the label to see if iron has been added.

Cereals aren't just for breakfast. Wheat, rye, oats, barley, corn and rice are all cereal grains. The products made from these grains are part of this group. Breads, crackers, macaroni, spaghetti and so on all belong here, too.

Cakes, doughnuts and cookies also contain flour, but they do not belong to the bread and cereals group because the amount of flour they contain is small. Choose small amounts of these "extras" and don't eat them often.

3. *Vegetables, fruits, legumes, nuts and seeds*

Vegetables and fruits give you vitamins, minerals and fibre. For example, folic acid and iron are needed to build red blood cells for you and your baby. Vitamin C is needed for strong teeth and gums. Your baby's teeth are made in the uterus, even though they don't grow in until after birth. Vitamin C will also help the absorption of iron when you don't eat meat. Vitamin A is needed for healthy skin and eyes, and for proper growth.

No one vegetable or fruit can supply all these vitamins in the amount you need. Some are sources of vitamin C while others are sources of vitamin A. Try to eat a variety of them each day. Include them in each of your meals. Take them as your preferred snacks. It's easier to think of fruit as a snack, but don't forget vegetables, especially those that are dark green or yellow. They may not be as sweet as fruit, but they generally contain more of the vitamins and minerals that you need.

Vitamins and minerals can be lost when you prepare and store foods. Cook vegetables for only a short time, using as little water as possible. Don't soak them.

Juices made from vegetables and fruits belong to this food group because they contain other good things, not just vitamin C. However, juices do contain less fibre than the fruit or vegetable they are made from.

Fruit drinks and punches, even those with added vitamin C, don't have many nutrients, so they are not included in this group.

4. Meat, poultry, fish and eggs

Foods in this group give us protein. You need protein to build and repair your body, and your baby's body needs protein when it is growing. You also get some iron and B vitamins from many foods in this group.

Because meat, poultry, fish and eggs contain very good protein, it is not necessary to have big servings. If your food budget is tight, meat does not have to be the main part of your meals. Have a small portion of meat with a larger portion of a starchy food. This way you will have more money for milk, vegetables and fruits, which are important too.

Some kinds of meat, such as spare ribs, the skin of poultry, weiners, bacon and most luncheon meat, contain less protein and also have extra fat. You don't need extra fat, even if you are pregnant.

If you have difficulty including meat in your menus, or if you are a vegetarian, there are some foods you can eat instead of meat to give you protein and iron. They are cooked dried beans, peas or lentils, tofu, nuts, seeds and peanut butter. Don't eat too many nuts or seeds or too much peanut butter. Although they are high in protein and iron, they also contain extra fat.

Extras

Foods in this group are cakes, cookies, sweets, chocolate, sugar, jam, sauces, butter, margarine, cream, snack foods and soft drinks. Many contain large amounts of fat, sugar and salt. Some contain a small amount of essential elements, but not enough to replace the food in the other food groups.

You eat these extras mainly for their flavour. They can be part of healthy eating if you choose them occasionally or if you take them in small amounts.

How much weight should I gain?

Most pregnant women should gain between 9 and 14 kg (20-30 lb.). The amount of weight you can gain depends on whether you weighed too much or too little before you were pregnant. If you are a teenager or are expecting twins, your weight gain may also be different. The rate at which you gain weight can be more important than how much you gain. You will want to gain about 1-3 kg (2-6 lb.) over the first three months. After that, you will want to gain about a kg a month (2 or 3 lb.).

If you are gaining too much weight, don't cut down on food from the four groups. Instead, cut down on the extras—cakes and cookies, french fries, ice cream and so on.

Pregnancy is not the time to diet or lose weight.

How much can I eat?

You do not need to eat twice as much food. You can usually trust your appetite to know if you are eating enough. After three months you will probably need about 2300 to 2400 calories a day, depending on how active you are.

What you eat is as important as how much you eat. Ask your doctor or nutritionist for a copy of *Canada's Food Guide.* This publication can help you see if you are eating enough of the major food groups. If you are eating too much food, cut down on extras, eat smaller amounts more often, choose low-fat foods, and cook your food with little or no fat. If you are not eating enough, choose more food from the four food groups.

When should I eat?
Start with a good breakfast, including food from at least three of the groups.

Some women find it hard to eat three big meals a day. You can eat smaller amounts four or five times a day, which may prevent upset stomach, heartburn or indigestion. Choose fruits, milk, cheese, juice or vegetables for your snacks.

What should I drink?
You will probably feel more thirsty than you used to. Drink six to eight glasses of fluids a day. Choose milk and water first, then juices and other fluids to add variety. Watch the amount of coffee, tea, cocoa and colas you drink. They are high in sugar or caffeine or both.

Plenty of fluids will help prevent constipation.

Do I need extra vitamins?
If you are healthy and you follow *Canada's Food Guide*, you probably don't need extra vitamins and minerals. Sometimes your doctor may tell you to take a folic acid supplement and an iron supplement because of the baby's needs and rapid growth.

If you were underweight or if you have special needs, you may also need a supplement. Talk to your doctor or nutritionist. Tell them about the foods you are eating. Find out if what you eat is low in folic acid, iron or calcium. It is better to get your vitamins and minerals from foods, but if you can't, a supplement may be recommended.

Some women don't drink enough milk. Maybe they are allergic to it, or they don't like it. A doctor may suggest those women take calcium. Remember that milk has many other things in it besides calcium. If you can drink milk or eat cheese or yogurt, that is better than taking calcium tablets.

Can food additives and preservatives harm the baby?

Additives and preservatives can be added to foods only after they have been tested and allowed by law. The list of ingredients on the label will tell you what has been added to foods. You can use the list to choose foods that have fewer additives.

Does it cost a lot to eat right?

There are ways to eat well without increasing costs. Compare prices. Plan your shopping trip. Include weekly specials in your menu. Choose foods from the four food groups and cut back on extras. Check to see if convenience foods really save time. Generally, the more cooking you can do, the cheaper it is. For example, it is usually cheaper to make your own spaghetti sauce than to buy it, but you have to have the time and energy to cook it.

If you want help with choosing, cooking and eating the right foods, ask a public health nurse or a nutritionist.

I am a vegetarian. What should I eat?

If you are a vegetarian and you eat eggs and milk, you can eat well for yourself and your baby. Check with a dietitian or nutritionist to be sure you are getting the right combination of foods.

What about alcohol?

Alcohol is a drug. It passes from your blood stream into your baby's. It can seriously harm your baby. No one knows how much alcohol is safe for a pregnant woman to drink. When you are pregnant, it's best not to drink any alcohol at all.

Just for partners

A good way to enjoy healthy eating is to share it with somebody in a pleasant atmosphere. Make meal preparation faster and more fun by working together on it. You are more likely to add extra vegetables if you are cooking for two or more.

Pack her a healthy snack or lunch when she leaves home for the day.

The best way to help is to eat well yourself. Both of you are going to affect the eating habits of your new baby. Why not begin right now and make healthy eating a habit for all of you?

Chapter 5

Daily Life while You're Pregnant

While you are waiting for the baby, enjoy yourself as much as you can. Look for ways to stay comfortable and relaxed. It is a time for you and your partner and any older children to enjoy being together, and to prepare a welcome for the new baby.

Sleep

As the weeks and months go on, your body will tell you to slow down. You will feel more tired and sleepy. Most people need eight hours of sleep a night; you may need more, or a little less. A nap or two during the day may be the best way for you to stay rested. Enjoy the time to rest. If you are always tired, tell your health care professional.

Work

Usually you will be able to keep working even in the last month of your pregnancy, if you want to. There is no need to stop working if you are healthy.

If your job is physically or mentally difficult, you may need to make some changes. There may be a way to switch to an easier job for a while or to work fewer hours; if you can't afford to work

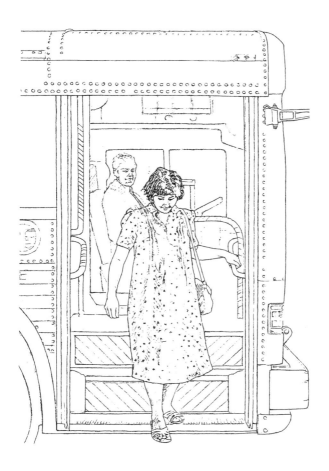

fewer hours, you may be able to get help with
money so you don't have to work so much.

You may have to switch to a safer job if you

work with dangerous chemicals or with machines that give off radiation that may be harmful to the developing fetus.

When you go out to work, don't get overtired. Try to rest for an hour during the day, or take a couple of shorter rests. When you come home from work, lie down for half an hour or an hour before you start to do anything. You won't have the same energy to work around the house. Maybe someone else will do some of the chores, or maybe some housework won't get done at all.

Try to put your feet up whenever you can, and don't stand and work. Standing is bad for the veins in your legs, especially if you tend to get varicose veins.

Try not to lift heavy things. If you have a toddler, you may be able to teach her to climb up beside you so you don't have to lift her up. Let someone else move the furniture around to make room for the new baby. Learn to lift and carry bags so you don't strain yourself.

Parental leave

Start now to explore the benefits available at your workplace. When you take time off to have the baby, you will have benefits under UI (unemployment insurance) at least. Ask your employer what additional benefits are available. Can you take an extended leave after the baby is born? Sometimes partners can get parental leave, too; you may be able to arrange your schedule so that you stay home with the baby for the first few weeks or months, and then your partner stays home for a time after you go back to work.

You may want to start to plan child care for when you return to work. See the section called "Day care while you work" in Chapter 15 for some ideas.

Daily physical activity

If you already have a sport, you can probably keep on with it. Continue swimming, curling, skating and so on. As your weight increases, your sense of balance changes, so it's not the time to learn downhill skiing, horseback riding or hard racquet sports.

Your joints are looser than they used to be, so running or high-impact aerobics are not good choices now.

If you don't get any other exercise, walk for an hour every day. Your body needs daily exercise to stay in good shape during the pregnancy. Exercise will make you feel good and help your body get ready to give birth to the baby.

Social life

Keep seeing family and friends as much as you enjoy them, but don't take on too much. It may be time to let someone else give the big party or have the family get-together this year. Avoid visiting where there are sick people who may pass something on to you.

Enjoy your social life, and pamper yourself. Come home when you are ready to. If you feel like an early night, give yourself a break.

Smoking

Smoking is bad for your health at any time, and it is bad for your baby's health. Both the nicotine in the tobacco and the carbon monoxide in the smoke will pass through the placenta into your baby's blood stream.

Nicotine makes the blood vessels close up so there is less room for nourishment to get through to your baby. If you smoke, your baby will be smaller and less mature than if you don't smoke.

Carbon monoxide in your blood means that your baby does not get enough oxygen. Lack of oxygen may cause damage to the baby's brain or eyes.

Women who smoke have a greater chance of miscarriage, premature birth, bleeding and other complications of pregnancy. Smoke is also harmful to children and other people around you.

Don't start to smoke. If you already smoke, cut down or stop. **It is never too late to quit.**

Travel

Car, train, plane or boat—travel as you like, but make sure you wear your seat belt or life jacket as required. After your thirty-sixth week, it is better to limit your travel since you could go into labour any time; try to stay near home. Airlines often limit travel for pregnant women in the last trimester.

Let someone else carry the heavy luggage, and plan your trip so you don't get too tired. Try to sit with your feet up. If you're in a car, stop every couple of hours to walk around a bit.

Avoid travel to places where there are no doctors or hospitals, or where there is an outbreak of disease.

Sex

Many women feel differently about sex during pregnancy. You may find your desires are different now; perhaps you are not so interested in intercourse, or maybe familiar positions are not comfortable for you any more. On the other hand, you might find sex even more enjoyable.

There are many ways to express your love physically. You and your partner together can figure out how to give each other pleasure in ways that suit your feelings and the changes in your body.

Sex shouldn't cause pain or make you feel uncomfortable. If there is an abnormal discharge, don't have intercourse until you talk to your doctor.

Baths

A shower or bath every day will help you stay clean and comfortable. You can take a tub bath all through your pregnancy if you like; the baby's temperature will not go up during a regular bath. As your balance changes, you may find getting in and out of the tub a challenge. An anti-slip bath mat or some stickers on your tub will make your footing more secure.

Saunas and hot tubs

Saunas and hot tubs are not recommended during pregnancy, because the high heat may raise your body temperature. This may endanger the baby, causing birth defects or even death.

Clothes

Wear clothes you feel comfortable in. If you start to wear a good bra as soon as you know you are pregnant, it will support your breasts as they get bigger.

Wear loose clothes. Garters or knee-high stockings, or anything tight around the legs, may make your legs swell or make varicose veins worse.

Some women wear panty hose and find them comfortable. Support hose may keep your feet from swelling. If you wear support hose, put them on before you get out of bed in the morning.

Comfortable shoes with low heels will help you keep your balance.

Douches

You won't need to douche to keep clean. A bath or shower, or washing yourself from front to back, will do that. If you have a lot of discharge, or if you get an infection, tell your doctor.

Drugs and medication
Don't take any drugs or medication without asking your doctor!

Some drugs can harm your baby, especially in the early months of pregnancy when the baby's body is being formed. Everything passes through the placenta to the baby. When you first see your doctor, tell him or her about all the drugs you are taking. Mention drugs prescribed to you and ones you buy over the counter in the drugstore or supermarket; if you use street drugs, tell your doctor about those, too.

Even drugs you took before you were pregnant, such as cold medicines, should be prescribed by your doctor when you are pregnant.

Drugs like heroin and cocaine are even more serious because the baby may be born addicted to them.

Stress

Things may bother you more than they used to, but you will find the same things that used to get you through the rough spots will work now that you are pregnant. Your sense of humour is high on the list of lifesavers. Laughing at the ridiculous things that go on is a sure way to relax, and sharing the joke is even better.

Get lots of rest and eat well. When you feel good, you can cope with whatever comes along. You may find your daily walk is a good chance to let off steam about what's bothering you.

Plan ahead. If you decide what is possible and what is impossible for you to do, you can make room for the really important things. When the important things are taken care of, it is easier to stop worrying about the rest.

Confide in someone you trust. When you are

worried, talking it out will release some tension and will often lead to a solution to the problem.

Around the house
You may have many spray bottles around your home—cleaners and air fresheners and insecticides and so on. Now that you are pregnant, don't use them. Be especially careful not to use oven cleaners, paint strippers, insecticides and other sprays that tell you to leave the house while they are working, or ones that must be used in a well-ventilated area.

Used cat litter sometimes has a parasite in it that can cause toxoplasmosis. Toxoplasmosis is an infection that is not harmful to you, but it can have very serious effects on an unborn baby. It may produce eye and brain damage, or cause your baby to be born prematurely. Let someone else change the litter box.

Most hospitals have a poison control centre. The staff will be happy to discuss your concerns about chemicals, drugs and other things that might be harmful to you and your baby.

Just for partners
Nine months of waiting for the baby gives you time to get used to the idea of an addition to your family.

Decisions about staying home with the baby, or about finding a day-care centre or a home day-care provider, are decisions for both parents to make. Do some of the legwork to find out what is available in your community so the two of you can think about it together.

Try to take stress off your partner by assuming responsibility for some of the household work; plan together so the important things get done, and agree about what isn't important, so no one will worry if everything isn't finished.

Your sense of proportion and your sense of humour are big assets at this time. You will probably look back later and laugh at things that you worry about now. If you can laugh now, this waiting time will seem to pass more quickly; a shared laugh can help cement a relationship.

Chapter 6

How To Stay Comfortable

As your body gets heavier, you may find it hard to carry the extra weight around, but exercise and good posture will help you keep fit and make you more comfortable.

What kind of exercise? It depends on what you're used to and what you like to do. There may be an exercise program for pregnant women in your community that will be just what you need. At your prenatal classes you will also learn some exercises to do now and during labour.

Exercising with your partner can be fun; if you work together now on the exercises, you will be comfortable working together during your labour.

Stand straight, sit straight
The weight of your baby pushes forward. If you keep your body straight and your back straight, you will feel better.

Head: Keep your neck straight.

Shoulders and chest: Lift up through the rib cage. Pull your shoulders back. Roll your arms out.

Abdomen and buttocks: Tighten your abdominal muscles so your back becomes flatter. Tighten your buttock muscles and tilt your hips back.

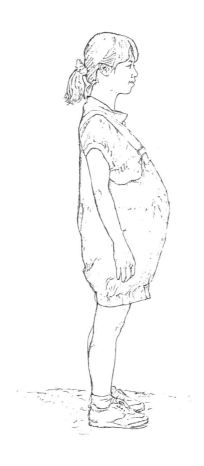

Knees: Bend your knees a little.
Feet: Keep your feet flat on the floor, and in
two parallel lines, turning out neither the toes nor

the heels. Put your weight on the middle of each foot, not on the toes or the heels.

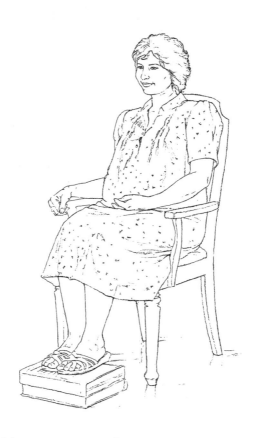

Making your muscles stronger
There are two groups of muscles that change a lot

when you are pregnant: the abdominal muscles and the pelvic muscles. As the uterus gets bigger, your abdominal muscles have to stretch to reach around it. The muscles at the bottom of your pelvis soften up to allow the baby to be born. These muscles are very elastic. They have to be able to stretch to let the baby out, and then return to normal after the baby is born. They get stronger and more elastic if you exercise them.

There are some exercises that can help you keep these muscles tight and strong. If you do them, you will not have so many backaches during pregnancy, and you will get your shape back more quickly after the baby is born.

Sometimes when you are pregnant, or afterwards, a little urine will be squeezed out when you cough or sneeze. You can stop the urine from leaking out if you tighten your pelvic muscles just before you sneeze or cough.

Tighten your pelvic muscles

This exercise is for the muscles around the vagina, rectum and bladder. It will help you control these muscles and help the muscles support your uterus and your other organs.

You can learn to do this exercise while you are sitting on the toilet. While you are urinating, tighten your muscles to stop the flow of urine. Relax and let it flow. Tighten up the muscles to stop it again. Relax.

Now you know where those muscles are. Tighten them up and relax several times a day.

You can do it sitting down or standing up. If you are standing, put your heels together and turn your toes out while you tighten your pelvic muscles.

Tighten your abdominal muscles

You can do this exercise when you are standing or walking, at the same time as you tighten your pelvic muscles.

Tighten up your abdominal muscles as much as you can. Hold them for a few seconds. Relax. Repeat this many times a day.

Relaxing

Relaxing conserves energy; it calms your mind, and reduces stress and fatigue. If you relax, a short rest will be enough to make you feel good again. Relaxation is a skill that will be useful all of your life, not just when you are pregnant.

If you learn to relax, you will feel less pain during labour. You will stay calmer and ready to do the work of delivering your baby.

How do you learn to relax? Here are some things for you to try.

Get comfortable. You can sit or lie down. Make sure all parts of your body are supported. Bend your legs and arms a little bit.

Once you are comfortable, make a tight fist with your hand. Start to breathe quietly and evenly. You will feel your fist start to relax.

Breathe your worries away

You may find that all your worries come rushing into your head as soon as you try to relax. Think about your breathing. Count your breaths as you take them. Or listen to something that has an even rhythm, like a clock ticking or some quiet music.

Close your eyes or keep looking at one spot on the wall. Focus on a happy thought or remember a happy place.

Relax your whole body

1. Tighten each set of muscles, then relax. Do one set at a time.

Left leg: Squeeze the toes down—relax. Bend the ankle down—relax. Bend the ankle up—relax. Straighten the knee a little way—relax. Tighten the buttock muscles—relax.

Right leg: Do the same as the left leg.

Left arm: Make a fist—relax. Bend your elbow a little—relax. Straighten your elbow a little—relax. Tighten the shoulder where you are lying on it—relax.

Right arm: Do the same as the left arm.

Face: Tighten up all the muscles of your face and neck, then let them all go loose.

Then tighten all the muscles you can. Hold for a few minutes, then relax all over.

2. When your whole body is loose, start to breathe with rhythm. Think about your breathing. Breathe quietly and naturally.

3. As you breathe in, say "in" very slowly. Then

breathe out and say "out" as you do it. Keep your mind on the "in" and "out." The words will keep your mind free of thoughts.

When you are totally relaxed, the floor will seem soft; you may feel it pushing you up. You may fall asleep.

When you are ready to get up, move around a bit first. Stretch your legs and arms, and sit up gradually. If you get up too quickly, you may feel faint or dizzy.

As soon as you can relax your muscles group by group, try to relax everything at once. You will want to be able to do this during labour.

Practise relaxing before you go to bed at night and before you have a rest.

Once you have learned how to relax, practise. You are learning to relax so that when you are in labour you can relax whenever you need to. You are going to be tense during labour, so practise relaxing now when you are tense or under stress.

Practise with your partner. Practise often.

Lying on your back

Early in your pregnancy, you may find lying on your back is a comfortable way to rest. Later you may feel dizzy if you lie on your back, because of the weight of the baby on the blood vessels.

You may want to put one pillow under your head and another under your thighs. Let your legs and feet roll out. Bend your elbows a little.

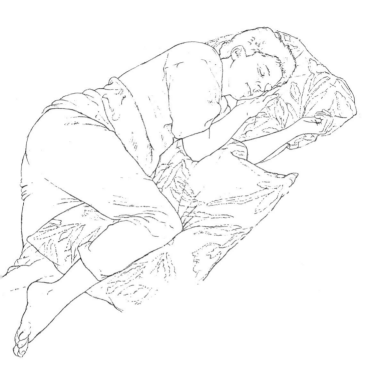

Lying on your side
Later in your pregnancy, and when you are in labour, lying on your side may the most comfortable position for you.

The picture shows you where to put your pillows. Bend your arms and legs a little bit.

Just for partners

If you are going to be her labour coach, go to classes with her and help her practise relaxing. Exercise together and relax together. Relaxation techniques may help you stay calm during labour, too. Sometimes it will seem like a long time to wait. Try to keep your sense of humour. If you can laugh together, the waiting time will be fun for both of you.

Chapter 7

Getting Ready for Your Baby

Getting ready for the baby is something the whole family can enjoy. It will make everyone look forward to welcoming him when he comes home from the hospital.

If you have children, this is a good time to talk about sex, sexuality and reproduction. They will love to look at their own baby pictures and baby clothes while you talk with them about babies, what they need and how they grow. It will interest them in the idea of a new baby, and may make them ready to love the newcomer and more willing to share you with him.

If you have to move your older child out of her room or her crib to make room for the new baby, do it now. Give your older child lots of time to get used to this new way of sleeping. If you wait until the new baby is home, the older child may feel the baby has displaced her, not only from her bed but from your attention.

What does a baby need?

Right now you need to get only a few basics—a crib, some clothes, some diapers, something to bathe the baby in, and a car seat. You can add things later if you think you need them. Safety is the most important point when you are buying things for the baby, especially if you are buying or borrowing secondhand equipment. For more about safety, see Chapter 16, "Safety and First Aid."

Crib
Your baby needs a safe place to sleep. Canada has very strict rules about crib safety; to be safe, don't buy or use any crib made before September 1, 1986. The date should be on the crib; if there is no date, the crib is too old and is not safe.

The baby needs a firm mattress to sleep on; if it is too soft, he may smother. The mattress should fit snugly into the crib. Try to put two fingers between the mattress and the side of the crib. If both fingers fit, the mattress is too small.

Never put a pillow in a crib, because the baby may smother in it. Never get a water bed for a baby or let a baby sleep on one. They are too soft, and the baby may not be able to breathe if he is sleeping on his stomach.

The crib also needs:
- bumper pads for the sides
- three to six quilted pads
- two rubber or plastic sheets
- six crib sheets
- three or four warm blankets

The baby's room should have sunlight, a window that opens, no drafts, and blinds or curtains so you can make the room dark when you want to. If you are going to keep the baby in your room, make a corner of it especially for him.

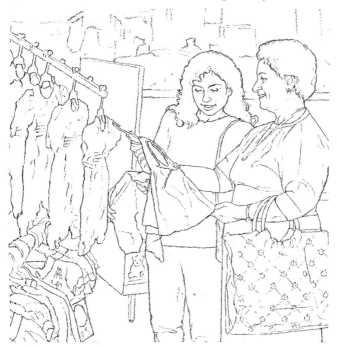

Clothing

Babies usually grow out of clothes before they wear out, so hand-me-downs from friends or family are wonderful. Look out for secondhand clothes, too.

Here are some things to think about when you are buying baby clothes:

- They should be big enough so the baby feels comfortable.
- They should be plain. Buttons or decorations

come off and the baby might swallow them.
- They should be easy to put on. Look for things that don't go over the baby's head, or that have big openings for the head.

What should you have? Six or eight T-shirts, six to eight nightgowns or sleepers, some booties and a couple of sun bonnets will do to start. Babies grow very quickly, so buy things in year-old sizes.

The baby should have his own washcloths and towels.

Whenever you get new clothes, blankets or towels for your baby, wash them before you use them. New things have lint on them, and there is also a special finish on new cloth that can bother a baby's skin.

Pack some diapers, a shirt, a nightgown, a blanket or shawl and a bonnet in a little bag. When you are ready to bring the baby home from the hospital, someone can bring the baby's things in to you.

Diapers
Diapers are a big item in a baby's wardrobe, and, since a baby wears diapers for more than two years, they will be on your mind for a long time. You have three choices: using a diaper service, washing cloth diapers at home, or using disposable diapers. How to choose? Here are some questions to consider:
- What is available in my area?
- What fits my budget?

- What is most convenient?
- What is best for the environment?

Cloth diapers

Cloth diapers have changed in the past few years. It used to be that they were square or rectangular pieces of cloth that had to be folded after each washing and were held in place with pins.

Now you can buy "prefolded" diapers made with thicker cloth in the middle, so they are not so bulky on the baby. And just coming onto the market are cloth diapers that are specially shaped to fit without any folding. You may have to buy a bigger size as your baby grows. Some have Velcro tabs instead of pins or come with special clips. If you use pins, buy the ones with metal closures, not plastic.

Plastic pants or cloth diaper covers can be used to keep the rest of the baby's clothes dry. Often the diaper covers are made of a fabric that "breathes." They keep the outer clothes dry, but air can get inside them to help prevent diaper rash.

Washing diapers at home: If you wash diapers at home, it will be cheaper than a diaper service but more work. Make sure the diapers are rinsed well. Add a cup of vinegar to the rinse cycle. It acts as a softener.

You will need at least twenty-four diapers to start with, but it will be more convenient if you have about three dozen.

Diaper service: A diaper service will bring

clean diapers to your door and take away the dirty ones. You just rinse the dirty diapers and put them in the pail; the service washes, dries and folds them, and brings them back.

Usually it is cheaper to use a diaper service than to buy disposable diapers.

As well, a diaper service may be better for the environment than washing at home. If a service is certified by the Environmental Choice Board and uses their label, it will use about half the water, energy and detergent that would be used to wash the diapers at home.

Disposable diapers

Disposables are convenient but more expensive. Although you can just throw them in the garbage, they take up a lot of space at landfill sites (dumps). They are made mostly of wood pulp and plastic; the pulp uses trees, and the process of making it causes air and water pollution, as does the manufacture of plastic.

Some makers of disposable diapers are looking into recycling programs to take care of some of these problems.

What else does the baby need?

You will save steps and aggravation by keeping together all the things you need to bathe and change the baby. You could use a tray or a cookie sheet or a basket to hold these things:

- mild soap in a dish
- covered jars for safety pins and cotton balls

- baby oil or Vaseline
- powder or cornstarch
- washcloths and towels

You will need a bath basin, or something large enough to bathe the baby in, and somewhere to store all these things.

If you are using cloth diapers, you will need a diaper pail to soak used diapers in.

If you are going to bottle-feed your baby, you will need:
- six large bottles (227 ml/8 oz.)
- two small bottles (114 ml/4 oz.)
- nipple caps and nipples

These are some other things you may want to think about getting later on: a baby carriage, a high chair, a stroller, a small potty, a toilet seat, a playpen and an infant carrier, either a front pack or a back pack.

Car seat
Buckle up. It's the law. You will need a car seat to bring your baby home from the hospital. Often you can rent or borrow one from a community group. See the section called "How do I keep my child safe in a car?" in Chapter 16 for more information.

Getting ready to go to the hospital
A month before your due date, pack your bag for the hospital. It will be ready for you to pick up and go any time. Put in it:
- nightgown

- housecoat
- slippers
- toothbrush, deodorant, etc.
- make-up if you wear it
- quarters for the pay phone
- a magazine, a deck of cards or something else to do

At home, keep these numbers beside your telephone:

- your doctor
- the hospital
- a taxi company
- the person who is going to look after your other children while you are away

Keep your health card with you.

Talk to the person who will drive you to the hospital. Be sure he or she knows the way. Find out which door to use at the hospital in the daytime and at night.

Sometimes you can register at the hospital before you go in. Ask at your prenatal class or at the health unit.

Feeding your baby

Now is the time to think about whether you will breast-feed your baby or feed him with formula. It's a big decision, and you will have lots of questions to ask your prenatal instructor, doctor or nurse. See Chapter 13, "Feeding the Baby," for more information.

Just for partners

Even before the baby is born, you can start to share his life. Prepare your home to welcome a new baby. Help figure out where the new baby will sleep and what he will need to make him safe and happy. You can share the decisions about what to buy for him.

If there are older children, talk to them about the new baby. Show that you welcome the new one, but that you still love them. Make time for the older children so they don't feel left out. How can the older children help you get ready for the new one? If they help, they won't be as jealous.

If you are going to be the birth coach, you will have an exciting part to play soon. Of course you are a little nervous. Talk about your feelings with your partner; let her know what you are thinking. If you are not sure what to do, ask lots of questions at the prenatal classes.

If you are going to drive her to the hospital, make sure you know where to go at any time of the day or night. Let your partner know you have taken care of some of the arrangements.

Chapter 8

Having Your Baby

As your due date gets closer, you may have only two things on your mind: "I want to meet this baby I've been carrying for so long" and "It will be great to see my feet again."

No one knows for sure when her baby will be born. A baby born anywhere from two weeks before the due date up to two weeks after the due date is considered "on time."

How can I tell it's getting close?

If this is your first baby, you may notice a change in your shape two or three weeks before the baby comes. The baby may move down in your body as her head gets into the birth position. This change, called lightening, will make your breathing easier and sleeping more comfortable. You may have to urinate more often because there will be increased pressure on your bladder. In later pregnancies, the baby may not move down until labour starts.

You will have cramps or contractions in your lower abdomen; these are called Braxton-Hicks contractions. Your uterus is complaining a little about being stretched. These contractions will not be regular, but you will feel them from time to time.

Your vagina will be wetter. The secretions will

soften the cervix so it will be able to open wide enough for the baby to be born.

Signs of labour

Labour starts differently for different women. You may have a backache that moves around to the front. If you put your hands on your abdomen, you can feel the uterus tighten.

You have a thick mucous plug in your cervix, which has been there throughout the pregnancy. Before labour starts, or early in the first stage, the plug comes out of the uterus, along with a little blood. You may see a pink stain on your underwear; this is called a bloody show. It is a normal sign and may happen a day or two before labour starts.

Your contractions will start. At first they may feel like period cramps, but short, weak and far apart. Slowly, they get longer, stronger and closer together. During labour they usually come in a regular pattern.

Talk to your doctor ahead of time about when to come into the hospital. When your contractions become regular or very uncomfortable, follow your doctor's instructions. If you are not sure, call your doctor or the hospital. Tell them what your contractions are like and how far apart they are.

Your water may break. This water is from the sac of amniotic fluid that has been protecting your baby in the uterus. The bag breaks before the baby is born. If your water breaks, go to the hospital, **even if you are not having any contractions.**

If you feel like it, you can have a drink of water or a light snack at this early stage of labour.

At the hospital

If you have visited the hospital with your prenatal class, the procedures will be familiar to you. Go to the admitting department where staff will welcome you to the hospital.

In the labour room, the nurse will ask you some questions, take your blood pressure, give you an internal exam, and listen to the baby's heartbeat. She will also take blood and urine samples to be tested.

In most hospitals your partner or coach will be welcome to stay with you during labour and delivery.

Labour and delivery

There are three stages in the birth of a baby. First, the cervix gets thinner and wider. When the cervix is open, the next step begins. The baby's head is pushed out of the uterus first, and the baby is pushed along until she is born. In the third stage the placenta is pushed out, along with the amniotic sac and the rest of the cord. This third stage is the shortest step of all.

How to breathe during labour and delivery

While you are in labour, you can use your breathing to calm you down and help you relax. **Try to**

breathe in through your nose. Breathe out through your mouth.

You want to stay relaxed. If you hold your breath, you will be more tense. Remember to keep breathing. You should practise now; then when you are in labour you will be able to breathe calmly and deliver the baby. When you practise, don't overtire yourself.

In the first stage of labour, you will want to breathe slowly. Your chest should go up and down slowly as you breathe in and out. You can also practise breathing quickly and lightly so your chest moves faster. A third way to breathe is deeply, so that your abdomen goes up and down.

During the transition between the first and second stages, you will need to pant lightly and blow out the air.

In the second stage you will need to push as you breathe. Do not practise pushing now. Wait until the time comes; the nurses will be there to coach you.

Between contractions, you should breathe normally and try to relax. If you relax you will save your energy for the next contraction. You will be calmer. You won't feel as much pain, and you will be able to do the work of labour.

Other ways to relax and control pain
Visualization will also help you relax. Focus on something outside you or on something in your imagination. Your coach may offer you guided imagery, in which you follow verbal suggestions to

keep your mind calm and focussed on something pleasant.

Massage or firm pressure from your labour coach may help you relax knotted parts of your body.

TENS (Transcutaneous Electrical Nerve Stimulation) is a device you control yourself. Using a low level of electricity, it stimulates your nerves to block the pain signals.

First stage

The first stage, the longest part of the birth, starts when your contractions follow a regular pattern. The contractions get stronger and longer and closer together. For the first baby it may take twelve to eighteen hours for the cervix to open wide enough to let the baby's head out of the uterus. In later pregnancies, this stage will probably be shorter.

During this stage you can walk around, or sit and talk with your coach, or watch TV, or do whatever is comfortable. Change your position as often as you like. Some women like to have their backs rubbed. Try to urinate often; if your bladder is empty, you will feel better.

At the end of the first stage, there is a "transition" to the second stage of labour. Transition can last up to an hour, as the cervix stretches over the widest part of the baby's head. You may sweat or shiver. Change positions to stay as comfortable as possible.

Now the baby's head is moving out of the uterus.

Second stage

The baby's head is in the vagina and will soon appear. You will want to push.

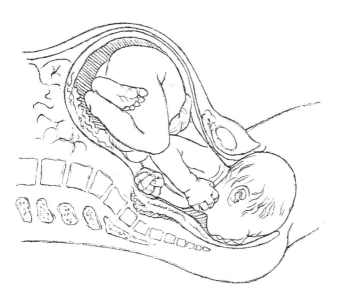

Many positions are used in the second stage. Find one that is comfortable for you. Women usually squat on the bed or sit up to push. The nurse and doctor will help you. Some women lie on their sides and push.

When you feel a contraction, take a deep breath. Then hiss or blow it out. Then take a quick deep breath and push. While you are pushing, let the air out with a grunting or moaning sound. Try to relax your pelvic floor, although it is very difficult. If your contraction is a long one, push for as long as you can. Then hold your breath for six seconds, take a quick deep breath and push down and out.

When the contraction is over, take a deep breath, let it out slowly and relax.

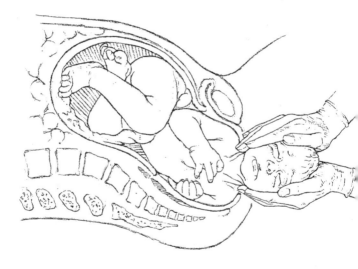

The baby's head will soon appear at the vaginal opening. There is a lot of pressure when the head is being born because it is the biggest part of the baby. If you push too hard, there will be too much pressure. The doctor or nurse may want you to pant so you will stop pushing. Take small shallow breaths and pant very quickly.

The doctor may need to make a small cut to let the baby's head out. This cut is called an episiotomy, and it will make the opening of the vagina a bit larger. You will not feel it being done. After the baby is born, the doctor will give you a local anesthetic and stitch the cut. If there is no episiotomy, there may be a small tear, which also will need to be stitched.

After the baby's head emerges, the doctor may use suction to clean out the baby's nose and mouth. Then the shoulders are born and the rest of the baby follows.

Baby is here
The hardest part is over. Your baby is here and may be laid on your abdomen. You may feel joyful, excited and tired all at once. If your partner is with you, you will be able to share your feelings with each other.

Third stage
After your baby is born, the uterus takes a little rest, followed by a few contractions. The placenta is then pushed out, along with some blood.

You will have some time to spend with your baby, to get acquainted and to bond with her. Then it will be time to get some sleep after your hard work.

Looking after the baby

The doctor will tie or clamp the cord, and the nurse will put drops or ointment in the baby's eyes to prevent infection. You and your baby will get name bands to identify you.

The doctor will check your baby's colour, cry, heartbeat, breathing, muscle tone and reflexes.

You will see the vernix on the baby's body, the creamy material that protects her skin. It will gradually rub off. While some babies look skinny and wrinkled, others are chubby. Some have blotches on their bodies. Your baby may be covered with hair, or she may have no hair at all. Every baby is different.

The baby's head will not be perfectly round because of the pressures on it during the birth. The head generally regains its shape within twenty-four hours.

Drugs during labour and delivery

Most women agree labour is hard work and sometimes it is painful. Relaxation techniques and working with your partner can help you get control and stay on top of whatever pain you feel. Some women want to have a childbirth without any drugs; others want to have some pain relief, and some don't want to feel anything. Talk to your doctor about what you would like. Don't wait until you are in the delivery room; at your regular visits to the doctor's office, be sure the two of you understand each other.

There is no perfect drug to take all the pain

away. Most drugs pass from the mother's blood stream into the baby's blood and make the baby sleepy; doctors and nurses will monitor the amount and timing of a drug to prevent the baby from getting too much of it, so she will be born alert and able to breathe easily.

As well, it is important that the mother be awake to do the work of labour; too large a dose of drugs for pain relief may rob her of the strength she needs to deliver.

Thirdly, it is important that mother and baby be alert after the birth so that the two of you can bond. The best time for this bonding to begin is right after birth.

There are four ways of giving drugs during labour:

Epidural: This is the most common. The drug will be injected into your lower back and you will feel numb from your waist down. Usually the doctor will let the drug wear off for the pushing stage, then renew it for the delivery. It doesn't affect the baby.

Pudendal block: A drug is injected through the vagina near the cervix to reduce the pain of the last contractions. It doesn't affect the baby.

Local anesthetic: Some doctors may use a local anesthetic to do an episiotomy, if needed, and to stitch it up. It doesn't affect the baby.

General anesthetic: A general anesthetic is rarely used unless there is an emergency.

Forceps and suction

Both forceps and suction can be used to help deliver the baby if the contractions are too weak or the baby is large. A forceps is a device shaped like two spoons that are placed around the baby's head; the doctor pulls gently with them, guiding the baby's head. If suction is used, the doctor will put a kind of a cap on the baby's head and attach it to a vacuum pump. It will be turned on during a contraction and will help the baby move down the birth canal.

Caesarean birth

You may hear this called a C-section. Sometimes the baby cannot be delivered through the birth canal and must be delivered through an incision in the abdomen. The doctor will give you an epidural or a general anesthetic.

For the first day after the operation, you may be sleepy; you may have some pain around the incision. You may have an intravenous (I.V.) tube in your arm and a catheter into your bladder. The catheter drains urine to relieve pressure and stop pain at the incision. The catheter and the intravenous tube usually stay in for a day or so.

If you have a caesarean birth, you may feel disappointed because you didn't have a vaginal birth. It is normal to feel this way; you missed something that you had planned and waited for during the better part of a year. You may feel cheated because you didn't get what you expected. You may feel sad and need extra attention and cuddling. Talk about your feelings to your partner, or the doctor or nurse, or to another mother who has had a caesarean birth.

If you have another baby later, you may still be able to have a vaginal birth, or you may have another caesarean. You can still breast-feed your baby after a caesarean.

The nurse will want you to do deep breathing, coughing and leg exercises while you are in bed. Activity will make you heal faster, so a nurse will help you to get up and walk around. Gas will make your incision uncomfortable; walking will help relieve the gas pains.

You will be offered medicine for pain relief as you need it. You may find it more comfortable to put a pillow over your abdomen when you have to cough. The incision should be healed in a few weeks, but it may still feel a little sore for a couple of months.

Induced labour

Sometimes the doctor may have to start labour if it doesn't start by itself. Or your labour may start on its own, but be very weak or never settle into a regular pattern. Other reasons for inducing labour are certain illnesses like diabetes or heart disease.

The doctor will give you medication to make the contractions stronger. The medication may be in the form of tablets or gel inserted into the vagina, or in an I.V. tube. Sometimes the doctor will induce labour by breaking the waters of the amniotic sac.

Induced labour follows the same pattern as other labour. Sometimes it is faster and stronger than labour that has not been induced. You may have the same pain relievers.

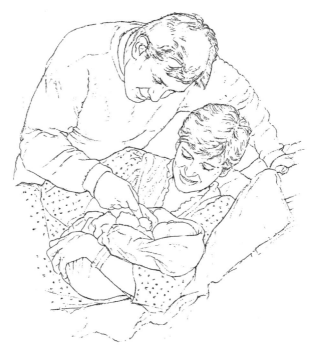

Just for partners
Your presence is a great help to the mother in labour. Just being there lets her know that you are in this with her. Be positive and calm. Talk with her and let her see your feelings. Respect her wishes.

Some women like their backs rubbed or their hands held; others don't want to be touched, but do want to be talked to.

Labour coaches have a lot to offer. The time you spent going to classes and practising breathing together will pay off now.

The time after the baby is born is special. You will find new ways to be together as a family.

Chapter 9

After Your Baby Is Born

After the birth of your baby, your emotions will be running high. You may show your happiness and excitement by crying or laughing, or you may be too tired to show any feelings at all. Certainly you will be very tired and hungry, and you will want to see your baby and hold him.

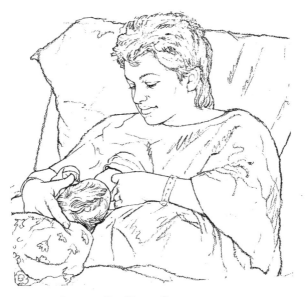

Breast-feeding after a C-section

Looking after the mother

Before you leave the delivery room, the staff will check your blood pressure and pulse. This is a good time to breast-feed your baby because he is usually wide awake right after delivery. Breast-feeding also helps firm up the uterus, which means there will be less bleeding. If you haven't had anesthetic, you will be able to move around easily. You may feel a little sore from the stitches, and you may be feeling afterpains. These are contractions that help the uterus shrink back to its usual small size.

How long will I stay in the hospital?

It depends on a lot of things. Some doctors favour a longer stay than others; hospital policy is different in different areas of the country. Partly it depends on the kind of resources your community has to offer. If there is a lot of support for new mothers at home, you may be able to leave the hospital earlier.

When you get home, remember that you can call your public health unit any time you want to ask a question.

While you are in the hospital, try to get lots of rest. You will probably want your family and friends to visit, but too many people will tire you out. Ask the nurse to make sure that your visitors don't stay too long. You need to sleep at night, and get two or three naps during the day.

These first few days are important for you and your baby. Your baby will be learning to trust you; you will be learning to respond to his needs. Make sure there is plenty of quiet time for the family to be together and to get to know each other.

If you have never had German measles, your doctor will likely recommend you be immunized against it. Since it is dangerous to have it done when you are pregnant, just after the baby is born is a good time for it.

You may feel sore all over—stitches, abdomen, breasts—and you may still be having afterpains. Ask the nurse or doctor for a pain reliever if you want one.

A warm bath will relieve the itchiness and soreness of your vaginal stitches.

If you had a caesarean, your abdomen will be sore for a few days; the incision will be sore too. Women who have had caesareans should shower instead of bathing until the stitches are healed.

More body changes

It will take about six weeks for your body to recover from the birth. Tissues heal in about ten days. During the first six weeks, muscles tighten up and the uterus goes back to its former size, about the same as a clenched fist.

The nurses will show you some exercises to help your body regain its strength and elasticity. Start to do them in the hospital and keep doing them after you get home.

How long will I need to wear a pad?

As your uterus sheds the lining that nourished the baby, you will have a discharge known as the lochia. For the first few days, the flow will be red. Then it will turn pink, and later brownish or yellowish white. You will need a pad for a few weeks.

It is important to keep the vaginal area clean so you don't get an infection.

- Wash your hands before you change your pad and again after you change it.
- Put on a clean pad every time you go to the bathroom.
- When wiping yourself or washing yourself, always wipe from front to back.
- Use a pad, not a tampon.

When will I get my period again?

Although this varies from woman to woman, mainly it depends on how you feed your baby.

If you use formula, your period will probably start between three and twelve weeks after the birth.

If you breast-feed your baby, your period will start a few weeks after you stop breast-feeding.

You can get pregnant again without ever having your period; this is a good time to think about birth control. See Chapter 10, "Planning Your Family," for more information.

My feelings are all mixed up

You may be feeling happy, sad, excited and scared, all at the same time. Many women find

that their feelings change a lot during the six
months following the baby's birth.

I cry for no reason!
Your mind is full of new experiences and your
body is full of hormones that make your moods
swing. Suddenly your baby is out in the world,
not inside you. The baby is a real person and
starts needing things from you right away. No
wonder you are tearful!

It takes time to get used to having a baby. Your
emotions will ebb and flow, changing suddenly
from happiness to misery. Let these feelings come
and go. Crying may help, and the day will come
when you will stop feeling so confused.

Share your experiences and your feelings with
other women who have had children. Talking
about it helps. Although every woman's experience
is different, you will have many things in common.

I can't believe it really happened!
There have been so many changes in such a short
time; sometimes it seems your body doesn't even
belong to you. You are very happy, but tired,
tired, tired. So much has happened, you may feel
unsettled. Although you are excited and happy,
you may still be confused and nervous.

You need someone who will listen while you
talk about everything that has happened. Talking
about it will make you feel more comfortable.
This unsettled feeling usually lasts for two or
three days after the baby is born.

I believe it! I believe it!

You start to take in what has happened. Your body feels like it might belong to you, at least sometimes. You want to know what's going on in your body, and you have lots of questions about your baby.

You want to look after your baby, but you feel that you need a lot of support. You may still feel nervous, not quite ready for all the new responsibilities. You are still tired, and little things bother you. You may feel that nobody wants you, that you aren't good enough to be a mother or a partner.

Your hormones make your mood change suddenly. You may be laughing one minute and crying the next. This stage usually lasts up to two weeks.

I can handle this!

Later, as you get used to the changes in your body, you start to feel more comfortable. You are still tired, but you understand what is happening. You are more confident and more relaxed. You can arrange your day to get some rest, get some things done, and leave some things undone. It feels right to make these choices. You feel more confident that you can look after things as an adult. You may feel that you want other people to notice that you are a good mother, even if you don't do things the same way as everybody else.

You start to think about getting back to your old life. What about going back to work outside the home? What about your sex life? The new baby seems part of the family; you feel that you can handle problems as they come up. It may take you six months or so to get through all these feelings.

Looking after your baby
The hospital will have a class to show you how to bathe, dress, feed and change your baby. If you have any questions, ask them now, while the nurse is there. Don't worry about feeling silly or stupid—every question is worth asking. There may be classes in parenting for mothers and partners.

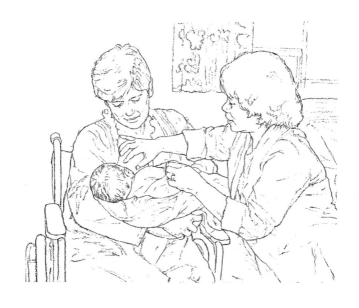

Rooming in or combined care

Your baby may stay in your room with you, rather than in a nursery down the hall. Most people like rooming in, because it seems more like home. The hospital staff will help you look after your baby. If you have practised in the hospital, it will be easier to look after him at home. Your baby will be used to you, and you will know what to do.

Some babies need special care

If your baby was born early or has special needs, he will need special care. So will twins or triplets.

A premature baby is a baby that is born a few weeks too early, or a baby that weighs less than 2.5 kg (5.5 lb.). It may be difficult for a small baby to stay warm, to breathe, to swallow and to digest food. He may get tired or sick more easily than a bigger baby. He needs special care until he gets bigger and stronger.

Occasionally babies are born with a birth defect. However difficult this is, there are people to help and support you. The baby may be transferred to another hospital. Ask for explanations of what is happening and what special treatment your baby needs. Your doctor should tell you right away, to relieve some of the confusion. If you are not familiar with these special needs, it will help to talk to other parents of children with similar needs, who have had to cope with the same things. Ask your doctor to put you in touch with someone to talk to.

My baby is in an incubator

Some babies can't keep themselves warm. They stay in an incubator, sometimes called an isolette. The isolette helps keep the baby's temperature even. It also makes it easy to give oxygen if necessary.

You can visit the baby, and talk and sing to him. You will likely be encouraged to touch him, because your voice and your hands are important to the baby. Check with the nurse about bringing soft toys to put in the isolette. Later, as the baby matures, the nurse will help you take the baby out of the isolette for a few minutes to hug and cuddle.

Sometimes you will have to leave the baby in the hospital when you go home. Be sure to get the phone number so you can call to ask how your baby is. It is hard to be separated from your baby without much chance to get to know each other, but visit him when you can. He will like to hear your voice and have you touch him.

Getting ready to go home
Help at home

This is an exciting time for you, but you will be tired; now that you have a new baby, you can't do everything you did before. Who can help? Your partner? Friends and family? Your other children? A friend or someone in your family might come and stay for the first few weeks, or come in every day to cook and do the housework.

Don't worry about getting everything done.

Enjoy your baby and let things go until you are back on your feet and feel like taking them on again.

Fill out those forms!
The hospital staff will give you forms to fill out. One form is to register the birth of the baby. Another form will notify the federal government to start sending you the family allowance for the new baby. The forms must be signed by someone who works at the hospital, so fill them out before you leave.

Birth control
Your doctor will give you a checkup before you leave the hospital and will ask you to come in for another checkup in four, six or eight weeks. Keep track of your questions so you can be ready to ask them at this next checkup. Birth control is an important issue at this time. You and your partner will want to discuss the timing of another baby, so that your body has a chance to recover from this pregnancy.

There are many different methods of birth control; you and your partner can find a way that is good for both of you. Chapter 10, "Planning Your Family," has more information. The nurses in the hospital or public health nurses can also answer your questions.

Part of the family
Whatever the shape of your family, a new baby

makes a difference. Make time for the rest of the family to get to know the new baby, to hold him, care for him and play with him. This is the time to welcome the new baby with love.

Just for partners
Visit the mother and baby, and participate in your baby's care as much as you can. The new mother will be anxious to have you make a good connection with the baby, and you will want to continue the bonding process that started in the delivery room. Holding and talking to the baby, and sharing your feelings with your partner, will help cement the bond.

If you have older children, you have a big role to play in helping them adjust to the changing situation. Take them to the hospital to see Mom and welcome the baby. Let them choose a present or make a card. This is a good time for a special outing with you.

New mothers need rest. If there are too many visitors, ask people not to come so often or stay so long. Offer to bring messages so everybody doesn't have to come every day.

With your partner, read the section above called "Getting ready to go home." Finalize your plans about help at home and put the plans into action. Fill out the forms. Discuss birth control.

If you share the work of planning for and looking after the baby, she will be able to relax and enjoy you both.

If your baby has special needs, share your

worries and anxieties. You may need to be involved with transferring the child to another hospital or making decisions about the child's care. Get all the information you can and share it with her.

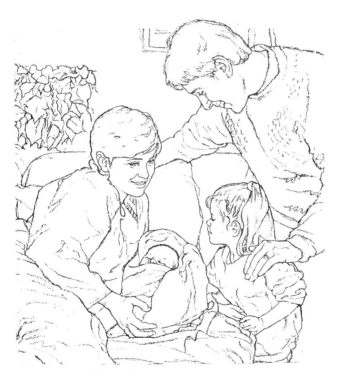

Once she's at home, pay attention to how she's feeling. If she can't eat, or if she won't get dressed, she needs medical help. Call the doctor yourself. Talk to your partner and find her someone else to talk to, too.

There are hormonal changes that may make her want to cry at the slightest thing. Let her talk to you about what's bothering her. Be patient. She will be more like herself soon.

Parents also want to do new things, have fun, socialize with other adults and meet their needs for love and sex. Although you may have less time and money than before, together you can make a plan to meet your own needs as well as the children's.

Something else you may have to tackle together is the problem of too much advice. It seems everyone has ideas about how to look after a new baby, and some of those ideas will be exactly opposite to what you have decided to do. If you and your partner have agreed about the way you will raise the baby, it will be easier to smile and say, "Isn't it interesting how many different ways there are to look after a baby?"

Welcome the baby into the family.

Chapter 10

Planning Your Family

After your baby arrives, give yourself some time to make her part of the family.

Before you are ready to have another baby, your body needs time to rest and heal itself. Your mind and spirit need to be rested and restored.

There are other reasons to use birth control. Your family may not be able to afford another baby, or perhaps you want to return to work. Maybe you think your family is already big enough.

There are many ways to prevent pregnancy. Birth control pills, the diaphragm and the condom are some common methods of contraception.

Each method has advantages and disadvantages. Some methods are better for some people than for others. You may want to change methods; sometimes one way is better, sometimes another.

Here are some questions to ask when you are thinking about each kind of birth control: Does it work? What side effects are there? How much does it cost? Is it easy to use? Is it comfortable to use?

There is information about many methods on the pages that follow. Talk them over with your partner. Take any questions you have to your doctor, your public health department or a family planning clinic. Get all the information you need to help you make a decision. Every couple must decide for themselves what kind of birth control they will use.

The birth control devices that are used by the woman are talked about first. Then there is information on devices used by the man.

Birth control pill

The pill works better than any other birth control device. Ask your doctor about possible side effects. The doctor will not give you the pill if you have phlebitis, high blood pressure or some liver diseases. When you are on the pill, you must see your doctor at least once a year.

The pill works because it stops the ovum, or egg, from leaving the ovary. If no ovum is released from the ovary, you can't get pregnant. Usually you take a pill daily for three weeks, then take none for a week. You will probably have your period during this week. You must take the pill every day at around the same time during the three weeks for it to prevent pregnancy.

I.U.D. (intrauterine device)

The I.U.D. is a very efficient method of birth control. It is a small piece of plastic that the doctor puts inside your uterus. It takes only a few minutes to insert. Then there is nothing else to remember, and nothing else to do. You will be able to feel the strings from the I.U.D. at the top of your vagina around your cervix. Check the strings every once in a while.

Some women cannot use the I.U.D. You should see the doctor at least once a year when you are using an I.U.D.

Vaginal diaphragm with spermicidal jelly or cream

A diaphragm is a rubber cup that fits over the cervix to stop sperm from entering the uterus. The diaphragm and a spermicidal cream work together to make sure the sperm can't reach the ovum.

A doctor will measure you for a diaphragm. After you have a baby, or if you gain or lose more than 2.5 kg (10 lb.), you should have your size checked; you may need a bigger or smaller one.

Before you insert your diaphragm, put about a tablespoon of spermicidal jelly or cream inside it. Spread a little of the cream around the rim.

You or your partner can insert it with your hands or with a special inserter. Then check to be sure it is in the right place. You should be able to feel your cervix through the diaphragm, something like feeling your nose through a rubber mask. Leave the diaphragm in for at least six hours following intercourse. If you have intercourse again during that time, put some more spermicidal jelly or cream into your vagina.

Vaginal spermicidal jelly, cream or foam

You can buy jelly, foam or cream at the drugstore. These products kill sperm. Use the plastic applicator to put them into your vagina just before intercourse. They are best used with condoms or diaphragm.

Vaginal sponge

A vaginal sponge prevents pregnancy in three ways. First, it contains a spermicide that is continually released into your vagina; second, it traps and absorbs sperm; third, it blocks the cervix so sperm cannot enter.

To use, take the sponge out of its package and wet it thoroughly with clean water. Squeeze it until it foams up completely. Fold it in half and insert it deeply into the vagina.

The sponge can stay in place up to twenty-four hours; leave it in at least six hours after intercourse. Take it out by gently pulling on the loop. It then can be discarded, as it should not be used more than once.

You can use the sponge while swimming or bathing, but do not use it during your menstrual period.

Fertility awareness and natural family planning

There are only a few days each month when you can get pregnant, around the time the ovum leaves the ovary and travels to the uterus. If you can figure out when your ovum leaves your ovary, you will know when you are likely to get pregnant. Both partners must be willing not to have intercourse, or to use birth control, on those days.

You can figure out when you are fertile by learning to watch for changes in your vaginal mucous or by using a special thermometer to keep track of your temperature.

This natural method requires both partners to know the times that you are likely to become pregnant. If you want to try this method, go to a birth control clinic and ask about it. Someone will teach you how to keep track of your fertile days.

Cervical cap
A cervical cap is a small rubber cap that the doctor fits over your cervix to keep sperm out. It is similar to a diaphragm and is available from some doctors.

Condoms
The condom is also called a safe or a rubber. It is unrolled over the penis just before intercourse. The sperm are trapped inside the condom and cannot move up the vagina.

Condoms work better when you also use vaginal spermicidal foam or cream or jelly with them.

Be careful when you take the condom off not to spill the semen anywhere in or near the vagina.

You can buy condoms in a drugstore or in a vending machine.

Condoms also help prevent the spread of sexually transmitted diseases (STDs).

Withdrawal

In the withdrawal method, the man takes his penis out of the vagina before he "comes" or ejaculates. It is not a good method of birth control because some sperm may come out of the penis before the man withdraws.

Sterilization

Sterilization is a permanent method of birth control. Women have a tubal ligation, an operation during which a doctor blocks the Fallopian tubes so that sperm can't reach a woman's ovum. Men have a vasectomy, where a doctor blocks the tubes that carry sperm. The man still ejaculates but there is no sperm in the semen (fluid).

Sterilization doesn't change how your body works in any other way. Both men and women can keep having the same sexual relations after they are sterilized.

Chapter 11

Getting Back in Shape

Exercise will get your body back to its old shape again by strengthening muscles, stimulating blood circulation and promoting healing.

You will start to do some of these exercises in the hospital. When you get home, keep them up. You will be able to do more exercise as your body gets back in shape.

Be sure to stand straight, sit straight and walk tall. Get lots of rest every day.

Pelvic tilt exercise

This exercise will stop backache and improve your posture.

1. Lie on your back.
2. Bend your knees.
3. Put your hand in the small of your back.
4. Tighten your abdominal muscles.
5. Push your back against your hand.
6. Hold and count to five.
7. Relax.
8. Repeat five times, increasing to ten times.

You can do this exercise sitting and standing, too.

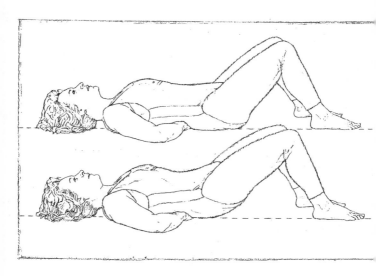

Sitting

1. Sit on a chair with your back against the back of the chair.
2. Tighten your abdominal and buttock muscles.
3. Push the small of your back against the chair.
4. Hold and count to three. Relax.

Standing

1. Stand with your back against the wall.
2. Put your heels five or six inches from the wall.
3. Tighten your abdominal and buttock muscles. This will press your back against the wall.

   Hold this position and walk around. Look at yourself in the mirror, and try to keep your body lined up like this all day. When you lift something from the floor, keep both feet flat on the floor. Bend your knees. Keep your back straight and lift the load in close to your body.

Pelvic floor contraction exercise (Kegel)

This exercise will help strengthen the pelvic muscles. It stimulates blood circulation, makes your bladder stronger and helps prevent your uterus from prolapsing (slipping) later in your life. Another result of doing this exercise is that your pleasure may increase during intercourse.

1. Lie on your back.
2. Cross your legs at your ankles.
3. Squeeze knees and thighs together. Tighten the muscles in your buttocks. Pretend you are trying to stop urinating.
4. Hold and count to five.
5. Relax.
6. Do it five times.

Later on, do the exercise without crossing your ankles. Do it sitting down and standing up.

Exercises for abdominal muscles

This exercise makes your abdominal muscles stronger, which in turn strengthens your back. As well, it helps you get into shape again.

Step 1 (Diagram A)

1. Lie on your back.
2. Bend your knees.
3. Put your feet flat on the floor.

4. Put your arms out towards your knees.
5. Push the small of your back to the floor.
6. Lift your head and shoulders. Keep your chin tucked in.
7. Hold and count to three. Later on, hold it for a longer time.

   Do it this way for at least six weeks, to give your body time to heal; then start to do the following variations.

Step 2 (Diagram B)
Do the exercise the same way, but start to sit up more. Instead of just lifting your head, lift your back and sit part way up.

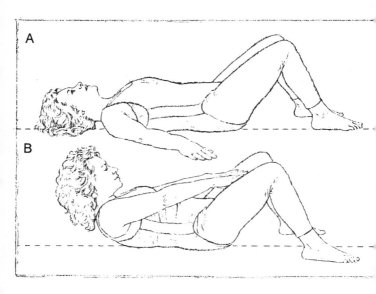

Step 3

This is the same exercise, except you use your arms to make it a little more strenuous. Do it like this:

1. Lie on your back.
2. Bend your knees.
3. Put your feet flat on the floor.
4. Push the small of your back to the floor.
5. Reach your right hand out to the outside of the left knee.
6. Hold and count to three and slowly move your hand back.
7. Do the same thing on the other side.
8. Do the exercise five times.

As it gets easier, increase the number of repetitions.

Chapter 12

First Days at Home

At last! You're ready to put your baby in her car seat and take her home.

Some things at home will be different because of the new baby, but don't change more than you have to. Your family has its own way of doing things, and keeping things as normal as possible will help everyone feel comfortable. The baby will get used to the way you do things, as long as she is warm and dry and well fed.

Don't worry if you have never taken care of a baby before. Your baby doesn't know you are a new parent. She will learn to trust you if you hold her firmly and lovingly. Accept her for what she is, and she will learn to accept herself. Let her know that she is safe with you and that you will take care of her needs. Your new baby is small, but she is tougher than she looks. She will soon get to know the family and will smile when she sees you.

Right from the start, your baby has a personality of her own. As you look after her and play with her, you will get to know her very well; you will be the "expert" on your baby. When you know what to expect of her, you will be able to tell when she seems to be sick or in a bad mood.

Baby's head

A new baby's head is big compared to her body.

Babies have one soft spot down the centre of the scalp and another one at the back of the head. Initially the soft spots are covered by a strong membrane, but bone slowly grows across them. The soft spot at the back closes by the end of the second month, the one at the top by the time the baby is eighteen months old.

Your baby won't be able to hold her head up until she is about four months old, because the head is too heavy and the muscles in the neck are too weak. Until then, use your hand to support the back of the baby's head when you pick her up.

Baby's face

Initially the eyes are grey or dark blue, but they will turn to their permanent colour in a few weeks or months. Babies can see as soon as they are born.

The baby may seem cross-eyed because she has trouble focussing at a distance. She will quickly learn how to do it.

Some babies have ears that seem to stick out too much. There is nothing you can do to make them lie flat. Putting a cap or a bandage on will not help. Later on, you can talk to your doctor about it if it still worries you.

Baby's legs

The baby's legs are not straight. They are a little curved because of the way she was lying in the uterus.

Baby's skin

There are different kinds of birthmarks that may appear on your baby's skin. Your nurse can explain them. These random marks are not caused by anything you did or ate while you were pregnant.

Baby's skin is soft, smooth and tender. Don't let it get cold or chapped. It is normal for the skin to peel a little. She may be covered with soft hair all over her body. This hair will fall out quickly.

Many babies get jaundice when they are a few days old. This makes their skin look yellow. If the colour gets more yellow after you go home, or if it turns yellow for the first time, call your doctor right away.

Some early changes

The baby's breasts may swell a little, and they may leak a little fluid. This is normal. Don't rub or squeeze them. If you rub them you may harm the nipple or cause an infection. The swelling will go down in a few days.

If you have a girl, her vagina may bleed a little, or there may be a white discharge. This is normal.

If your baby is a boy, his scrotum may be swollen.

When you change the baby's diaper in the first two or three days you will notice the bowel movement is very dark. Over the next few days it will change from tarry black to green to yellow.

Baby learns to trust

If your baby is hungry or cold or wet or in pain, she will cry to tell you she needs something. If you come when your baby cries, she will learn to rely on you to give her what she needs; she will learn that the world is a safe and welcoming place.

Cuddle your baby to let her know you love her and want her. Everyone in the family should hold the baby; sing or talk to her to make her a part of the family. Soon she will show you she is happy to be with you.

Sleeping

Your baby may sleep a lot for the first month or so, perhaps waking up only when she is hungry. If she falls asleep while you are feeding her, you can wake her by rubbing her feet, moving her around a little or stroking her cheeks. Some babies don't seem to need much sleep and stay awake a lot of the time.

While she is awake, let her spend time with people. Let her get used to being held and talked to. This will help her grow stronger, and it is good for her emotional development. You can protect her from getting too tired or too excited, but let her be part of the gang. She will want to be with people, and she will start to learn how to get along with people.

Crying

Your baby cries when she wants to tell you something. Is it time to feed her? Is her diaper wet or dirty? Maybe she is just lonely or bored. Bring her out where the action is. She will be interested in whatever is happening.

She may be crying because she is too hot or too cold. In the summer, dress her lightly and loosely. If her skin and head are damp, she may be too hot.

If her hands and feet are a little blue, she may be too cold. Our bodies adjust easily to a sudden change in temperature, but a baby's body cannot handle it. Help her adjust by adding or taking off her clothing. Think of her as a miniature you.

Soon you will know what your baby means when she cries. She will sound different when she cries for food than when she is lonely or sleepy.

Looking after the cord

Right after the baby is born, the cord is a bluish-white colour. It dries up, gets darker and falls off by itself, usually when your baby is one to three weeks old. When it falls off, there may be a raw spot, which may bleed a little. You can clean the bottom of the cord with a cotton swab dipped in rubbing alcohol. The alcohol also helps the cord dry up. The alcohol doesn't harm the baby, but it feels cold, and she may cry a little. Clean the bottom of the cord like this two or three times a day, or every time you change the diaper.

If your baby boy has just been circumcised, be sure not to get any alcohol on the circumcision.

Keep the cord dry while you give your baby a bath. When you diaper the baby, fold the top of the diaper down so the cord is outside. That way

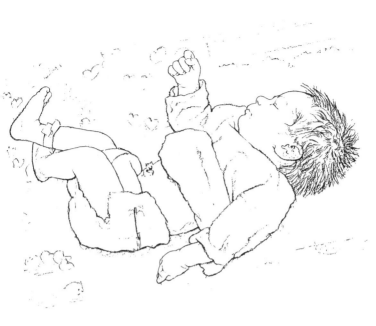

the air can dry it out. Usually you do not need to give it any special treatment.

Quite often the bellybutton sticks out, then turns in by itself. If you see some drainage from the bellybutton, if the skin around it turns red, or if there is a bad smell, there may be an infection. Call your doctor right away.

Bathing
You may feel clumsy the first time you give your baby a bath, but you will get lots of practice. Bath time is a good time to have fun. As the baby gets older, she will want to play and exercise more and more at bath time.

Choose any convenient time to bathe the baby, except right after a feeding. Don't bathe a hungry baby, either, because she will howl. It will not be a pleasant experience for either of you.

If the baby is having a hard time settling down in the evening, a bath may be a good way to calm her and make her ready to go to sleep.

You don't have to bathe the baby every day, but do clean the folds in her skin every day. There are folds at the top of the legs and arms, on the neck and elbow and at the back of the knees.

Keep the baby safe in the bath

- Don't leave your baby alone on the table or in the bath. When you reach for something, keep one hand on the baby.
- Don't add warm or hot water to the bath while the baby is in it.
- When you pick up the baby, hold the two heaviest parts, the head and the hips.
- Don't let anyone else use the baby's towel and washcloth.

Getting ready for the bath

Here is what you will need:

- basin
- soap—use a mild soap with no perfume
- towels
- washcloth
- hairbrush with soft bristle
- comb
- clean clothes and a clean diaper

The room should be warm, with the doors and windows closed to prevent a draft.

Take off your watch and rings or any other jewellery with sharp edges that might scratch the baby. Wash your hands. Make sure everything you need is beside the basin.

Fill the basin with lukewarm, not hot, water. Use your wrist or elbow to test the temperature of the water. If it feels comfortable, it is right for the baby's bath.

Don't interrupt the bath to answer the phone or the doorbell. Let them ring.

You can give your baby a sponge bath or a tub bath. Some hospitals and doctors recommend a sponge bath until the cord has fallen off.

Sponge bath

Bathe the baby quickly, so she does not get cold.

Eyes: Clean the eyelids with a washcloth wet with clear water. Start from the inside corner of the eye. Use a different part of the washcloth for each eye so you don't spread any possible infection to the other eye.

Face: Use the washcloth and clear water, no soap.

Nose: Don't use a cotton swab (Q-tip) to clean the nose. It could push mucous farther up into the nose and cause trouble there.

Ears: Wash behind the ears. Dry the outer ear and behind it. Don't use a cotton swab, or anything with a point, to clean inside the ear. Any wax that is there will come out by itself. If you try to get it out, you will only push the wax farther inside the ear, which could be harmful.

Hair: The baby's hair needs to be washed only once or twice a week. Wrap the baby in a towel or baby blanket and hold her under your arm like a football. Hold the baby's head over a basin or tub with her face turned up, and, using a mild soap or baby shampoo, wash her hair gently. It is important to rinse well because leftover soap will dry the skin out. After you have dried the baby's hair, brush it gently.

Care in washing and rinsing her hair will generally prevent cradle cap, a condition in which the baby has white flaky crusts on the scalp.

Cord: Keep the cord as dry as you can.

Body: Wash the body with your hand or a washcloth, starting at the neck and working down. Be sure to clean the wrinkles in the neck and armpits and at the top of the legs. Turn the baby over and wash her back. If you use soap, be sure to get it all off.

Baby's bottom:

Girls: Wash gently from front to back. Then wash the rectum, also from front to back. Washing from front to back prevents germs from the rectal area getting into the vagina.

Boys: Wash and dry the scrotum and the penis. Do not push back the foreskin. Wash and dry the rectal area.

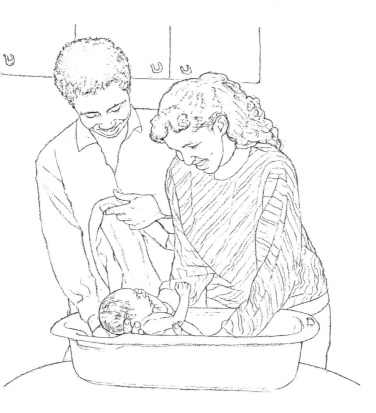

Tub bath

Fill the baby's bath with warm water to about 8 cm (3 in.). Use your wrist or elbow to make sure the water is not too hot or too cold. Slowly lower the baby into the tub, holding her with both hands and supporting her body with one of your arms. As you bathe her, keep a firm hold with one hand.

Wash the baby in the same way you would for a sponge bath, being careful to clean the wrinkles. Rinse all the soap off, then lift the baby out of the tub. Dry her quickly with a large towel. Check the folds of the skin to see if they are red or sore. Dry these parts very well.

Wash baby's hair as described above.

Dress the baby quickly.

When the baby is small, you can cut her fingernails and toenails after her bath. When she gets older, it is easier to cut them when she is sleeping.

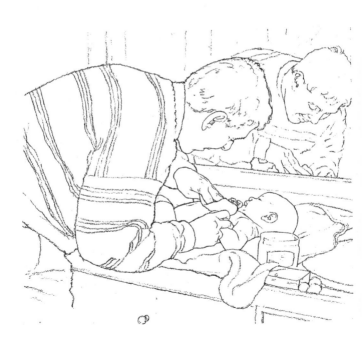

Clothing

A little baby needs only a shirt, diaper, night-gown or sleepers and a soft warm blanket tucked around her. In the wintertime, small babies wearing nightgowns need socks or booties. Give her a clean shirt at least once a day, or whenever hers is wet.

Cover her loosely so she has room to move around a little, and straighten her clothes and blankets so nothing is crumpled up under her.

Change her diaper before or after a meal, after her bath and any other time you have her up and she needs to be changed. If she wets her diaper when she is asleep, don't wake her up to change her. Wait until she wakes up.

Just for partners

Work out a plan together about how you will share the feeding and care of the baby. Who will get up in the middle of the night when the baby is hungry? Some couples take turns; in other homes the mother never gets up at night. If the mother is breast-feeding, she could stay in bed while you bring the baby to her and put the baby back to bed at the end of the feeding. If she is not breast-feeding, you could give the baby her bottle.

Either partner can bathe the baby, change diapers, dress the baby, do the laundry and so on. It is a shared responsibility. Both of you will want to cuddle the baby, play with the baby and comfort her if she is sick or out of sorts.

If there are older children, they need special

attention so they will feel good about themselves and the new baby. Help them do something special for the baby and their mother. Encourage them to talk to you about their feelings. What activity could you do with the older children that would be fun for all of you and reinforce their feelings of importance in the family?

Of course, the adults in the family need some time together too. Arrange a sitter so that the two of you can go out for a few hours.

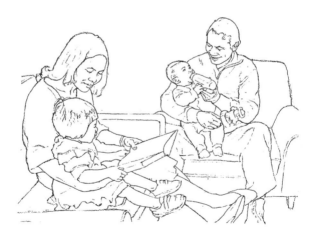

Chapter 13

Feeding Your Baby

Whether to breast-feed or bottle-feed your baby is a personal decision that should not be made lightly. Before making up your mind, learn about each method. What are the advantages and disadvantages? After gathering the facts, you and your partner can make the right decision for you.

Why breast-feed?

Breast milk is the most balanced food you can give your baby. It is never too rich or too thin. The antibodies in breast milk mean the baby is less likely to develop allergies. Breast milk is easier to digest than formula, so your baby is less likely to have an upset stomach or diarrhea.

Breast-feeding helps the uterus return to its normal size. It allows the mother and baby to have a special relationship with each other.

Breast-feeding is cheaper than using formula. You don't have to buy, mix, sterilize and store formula, bottles and nipples. It is generally more convenient, especially when you take the baby out, because you don't have so many things to carry.

Bottle-feeding

If you have chosen to bottle-feed, you and your baby can still have close times during feeding.

Use a commercially prepared infant formula.
Your doctor or nurse can help you choose the
best one and will tell you when to change to
cow's milk.

If you are away from home part of every day,
you might want to breast-feed your baby a
couple of times a day and bottle-feed when
you're not at home.

The next few pages are about breast-feeding.
For more information about bottle-feeding, go
on to page 136.

Breast-feeding your baby
How should I hold the baby?
Make yourself comfortable. You can lie down or
sit with your feet up. If you sit up, put a pillow
on your lap for the baby to lie on.

Hold the baby close to your body, skin to
skin, tummy to tummy, with his face level with
your breast and his mouth to your nipple. Don't
let him pull your breast down. Put his mouth a
little under the nipple so that his chin touches
your breast just below the dark part.

The baby should suck on the dark part of your
breast around the nipple, not on the nipple itself.
If the baby's lips are puckered up, he is sucking
only on the nipple; you will be sore, the baby will
get tired and less milk will come down. If the
baby is in the right place, sucking will usually not
hurt you, but you will feel pressure. If it hurts or
pinches, take him away from the breast and start
again.

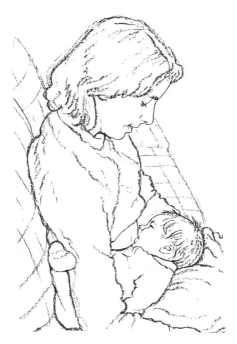

When your baby feels the breast, he will open
his mouth wide and feel for the nipple with his
tongue. When it touches the nipple, his lips will
close over the whole dark part of the breast. The
baby will seal it off with his mouth so no air can
get in. Then the baby will start to suck.

Is the baby getting any milk? If it is hard to pull
him away from the breast, he has made a seal with
his mouth, and he will be getting milk when he
sucks. You should hear him swallow and see the
sucking motion along his jawline up to his ears.

When you want to change breasts, put your

clean finger into the corner of the baby's mouth. This will break the seal, and it will be easy to move the baby away from the breast.

If you had a caesarean birth, you may be more comfortable if you lie on your side to breast-feed. If you sit up to feed the baby, put a pillow on your stomach. You might want to use the "football hold" to feed your baby. Support the baby along your arm against your side.

How often should I breast-feed?

Feed your baby every two or three hours at first, whenever he is hungry. The more your baby sucks, the more milk you make. It may take a few weeks for the two of you to establish a regular pattern of nursing.

I get cramps when the baby is nursing

When your baby sucks, you will feel afterpains for a few days. These contractions mean your uterus is going back to its old shape. If you have other children, the cramps may seem stronger with each child. You may have more vaginal flow.

Is my baby getting enough milk?

You can't see how much milk the baby is getting, but you can tell if it's enough. Your baby should have six to ten wet diapers a day and regular bowel movements.

Feel your breast after a feeding. It should be softer than before the feeding.

Your baby should suck hard at first, then settle

down, and may even go to sleep in the middle of or at the end of a feeding.

Is your baby gaining weight? Your baby will lose a little weight right after he is born, but he should gain it back by the time he is two weeks old. If he continues to gain weight, he is getting enough milk.

Keeping it up

If things are calm around you, and if you have enough quiet time to feed your baby, especially at the beginning, breast-feeding will likely be a good experience for you and your baby. Get into a pattern for taking care of your baby, and try not to break your routine.

- Rest as much as you can. Sleep when your baby sleeps.
- Drink a glass of water, juice or milk while you breast-feed.
- Eat a couple of snacks between meals.
- Let the baby nurse every two or three hours during the day and when he wakes at night.
- Ask your nurse or your partner to make sure you don't have too many visitors. Keep visits short. Give yourself time to breast-feed every two or three hours.
- At home, get help with the housework and cooking, so you have time and aren't too tired to breast-feed.
- If you have other small children, this is a good time for storytelling, listening to music and doing other quiet things together.

Bowel movements

If you breast-feed your baby, his bowel movements will be different than if you give him formula. For the first few weeks, your baby will often have a dirty diaper. He may have a bowel movement while he is feeding and again after his feeding. The stool is a yellow colour, or sometimes green. It will be very soft and watery.

Later, when he is two to four weeks old, his habits may change. He may not have a bowel movement for a day or two; he may have a bowel movement only every three to five days. So long as the stools are soft, the baby is not constipated, and there is nothing to worry about.

If you are feeding the baby formula, his bowel movements will be more formed and less frequent, and they will smell stronger.

Can I keep breast-feeding after I go back to work?

Yes. After the first few weeks your milk supply gets regular, and you can express milk manually or mechanically for feeding throughout the day. The caregiver can give the baby your milk in a bottle while you are at work. You can express your milk, store it in a fridge at work and bring it home with you.

You might want to breast-feed before you go to work, when you come home in the evening and before the baby goes to bed. The baby can have either your breast milk or formula while you are away. If you are going to mix formula with breast-feeding, it is best to wait until the baby is at least eight weeks old. By that time, your body will be making enough milk and your baby will be used to the breast.

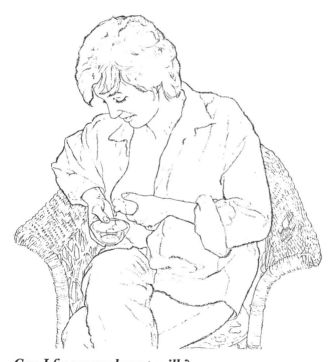

Can I freeze my breast milk?
Yes. You can express your milk and save it for sometime when you are away from your baby. If you are going to use the milk within twenty-four

hours, keep it in the fridge.

You can keep it in the freezer part of the fridge for two weeks. If you want to keep it longer than two weeks, it must be quick-frozen in a chest freezer and kept at -18° C (0° F). You can keep it in the freezer for up to six months.

Each time you express your milk, put it in a separate container. It is preferable to use sterile plastic bottles or plastic nurser bags. Close the bags with twist ties.

Put a label on every bag or bottle. Write the date on the label.

How to use frozen breast milk
Use the oldest bag or bottle first. Don't use milk that is more than six months old.

- Put the bag or the bottle under the tap and turn on the cold water. Let the water run until the milk in the bag starts to melt. Then put the bottle or bag in warm water until it is all melted. It should take about fifteen minutes.
- Never thaw the milk by letting it sit out in the room.
- Put the milk in the fridge until you are ready to use it.
- Some cream may come to the top of the milk. Shake it up a little before you use it.
- Use it within twenty-four hours. Throw out any milk that you don't use in a day. **Do not freeze it again.**
- *Do not use a microwave oven to thaw or to warm breast milk.*

Can I breast-feed my twins?

Yes! Many mothers of twins breast-feed their babies. Some mothers give the babies only breast milk; some also give a bottle of formula. Mothers of triplets, or even quadruplets, can breast-feed their babies.

You may choose to breast-feed both babies at each feeding or to breast-feed one baby at a time and give the other a bottle of infant formula.

Let your babies nurse often to encourage milk production. This means nursing your babies eight to ten times every twenty-four hours. If your babies are born early, and they stay in the hospital, you can express your milk and take it to them in the hospital.

My baby came early. Can I breast-feed?

Yes. Premature babies may not be able to suck at all or may not be strong enough to suck for very long. At first you can express your milk and the nurses will feed your baby with a tube.

How long should I nurse my baby?

You may choose to nurse for a number of weeks, or up to twelve months, or even longer. Let the baby give up the breast a little at a time; it will be easier on both of you. When you are ready to wean your baby, start with one feeding a day. Don't give the baby the breast at this feeding; instead give him formula by bottle or cup depending on his age. Do this at the same feeding time every day for a few days. Your body will make less milk as the baby drinks less from you. Then cut out another feeding. Give the baby formula at this feeding every day for a few days. As you cut down on breast-feeding, you won't need to drink so much liquid. Cut out a glass of water or juice a day each time you cut out a feeding.

Talk to your doctor or public health nurse if this is your first baby.

Support groups

If you have questions about breast-feeding, be sure to ask for help. You can ask the nurses in the hospital, your doctor or your public health nurse. La Leche League is a group interested in helping mothers to nurse their babies. In Quebec there are breast-feeding coaches (*marraines d'allaitement*) who will help you. Your doctor or nurse can help you find any of these groups.

The next part of this book is for people who are giving their babies formula. If you are breast-feeding, turn to page 128 for more information about feeding your baby.

Bottle-feeding your baby
Infant formula

Talk to your doctor or the nurse about what kind of formula to buy.

There are three types of formula:

Ready to serve: The formula is ready to use just as it comes out of the can. This is the most expensive kind.

Concentrated liquid: You mix it half and half

with boiled and cooled water before you feed it to the baby.

Powder: You mix the powder with boiled and cooled water, following the directions on the package. This is the cheapest kind of formula.

No matter what kind you use, it is important to measure exactly and to follow the directions carefully. If you add too much water, the baby will not get enough calories. If you add too much powder or liquid, the baby's food will be too rich and may make him sick.

Some formulas disagree with some babies for many different reasons. Your doctor may suggest you change formula if your baby develops a rash, cries a lot or throws up whole meals. No matter what kind of formula you use, you must keep everything clean. Germs grow quickly in formula; they can make the baby sick.

Making the formula

There are four steps to making formula: **Wash. Sterilize. Mix. Store.** Each step is important.

1. Wash
- Wash your hands.
- Wash everything well. Make sure there are no milk rings on the bottles; squirt hot water through the nipples to make sure the holes are clear. Rinse everything with hot water.

2. Sterilize
For the first three or four months, you must ster-

ilize the bottles, nipples and nipple covers to kill all the germs on them.

- Use a big pot that has a tight lid. Put a rack or a folded towel on the bottom.
- Punch holes in the lid of a jar big enough to hold all the nipples and the baby's soother. Put the nipples and the soother inside and close the lid.
- Lay the bottles on their sides in the big pot, but stand the jar of nipples up. Cover the bottles with water, but do not cover the jar. Steam will sterilize the nipples, and they will last longer than if you boil them in water.
- Heat the water until it starts to boil. Let it boil for five minutes and then cool.
- Handle everything you have sterilized with sterilized tongs.

3. Mix the formula

- Boil water for five minutes and cool it.
- Read the directions on the formula.
- Measure the formula and mix it with the boiled water.
- Pour it into the sterilized bottles. Put the nipples and the nipple guards on the bottles.
- If you are using a disposable nursing system, wash and rinse the holder well. Put a sterile liner in the holder; be sure you don't touch the inside of the liner. The nipples and caps must be sterilized before use, but it is not necessary to sterilize the holder.

4. Store

- Put the bottles into the fridge to cool down. Don't let them sit out, because germs grow quickly in warm formula.
- Keep them in the fridge until you are ready to use them, but make sure to use them within twenty-four hours. Never leave warm formula in a thermos or a bottle-warmer.
- If you are using powdered formula, keep the can tightly closed in a cool dry place. Use it within a month of opening it. If you are using liquid formula, keep the can covered and in the fridge after you open it. If you don't use it all within forty-eight hours, throw out what is left.

Warming the bottle

Warm the bottle in a pan of hot water or an electric bottle-warmer for a few minutes. Try a few drops on the inside of your wrist. It should feel neither hot nor cold.

Microwaves are not good for warming bottles. They work too fast; they may get too hot, and they do not heat the milk evenly. Some parts will be cold, while other parts will be too hot and may burn the baby's mouth. If you use too much heat, vitamins will be lost.

Feeding the baby

Sit up comfortably and hold the baby while you are feeding him. Keep the bottom of the bottle higher than the nipple to make sure the baby gets milk and not air when he sucks.

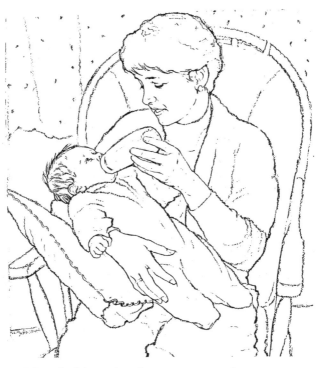

Most babies take about twenty minutes to drink a bottle of milk. Some babies take up to forty minutes, while some babies only need five minutes to get full. Throw out whatever formula is left in the bottle at the end of the feeding.

There are several reasons why you should always hold your baby to feed him and not leave him with a propped bottle:

- The baby may choke on the formula if he is lying down.

- You both miss out on a special relationship if you don't hold him while he nurses.
- Some studies show that ear infections are connected with putting the baby to sleep with a propped bottle.
- If your baby goes to sleep with a propped bottle of formula or juice, he may develop serious dental problems, beginning with cavities in his upper teeth.

What about burping?

A baby burps to let the air out of his stomach. When he is ready to be burped, he will slow down his sucking and may squirm a little. Probably he will want to burp soon after he starts to feed, in the middle of the feeding, and at the end. Some babies burp easily, while others don't.

There are several ways to hold the baby to burp him. You can sit him up on your lap, supporting his head. You can lay him on his stomach across your lap. Or you can hold him against your shoulder, supporting his head; then pat or rub his back.

Cover your clothes with a cloth in case he spits up a little.

Teaching your baby to use a cup

When your baby is about ten months old, give him a cup with some water or juice in it. He will learn to drink from a cup, and he will still be getting all the nourishment he needs from breast milk or formula. Soon he will be able to drink from a cup.

If he is on formula, you can let him have a cup instead of a bottle whenever he wants it. Most babies like a cup better by the time they are about a year old. Many babies will drink from a cup most of the time but still want a bottle sometimes.

Does my baby need water?

Sometimes your baby may be thirsty and will take a bottle of water, especially if it is hot outside, or if he has diarrhea or a fever. Babies who drink formula may accept water more often than babies who are breast-fed. If your baby is one of those who will never drink water, don't worry about it.

Do I have to boil the water for the baby?

Yes, until the baby is three or four months old, boil the water for five minutes. You can keep it in the fridge for two or three days in a sterilized container with a lid. Your baby will like water at about body temperature. When the baby has finished his bottle of water, throw out whatever is left.

What kind of water should I use?

If you are on city or town water, use the water from your tap.

If you have your own well, be sure the water is safe to drink. If you need information about getting your well water tested, ask your public health nurse.

If you are not sure the water is safe, or if you can't boil the water, you can use bottled water. Read the labels. You can give your baby "spring water" or "treated, non-mineralized water." Don't give your baby any other kind of bottled water, such as mineral water or Club Soda. Never use water from a lake or river or spring.

If you have a water softener attached to your tap or to the water hookup, the water may be harmful to the baby because of the extra salt the softener puts in it.

When to introduce cow's milk

Regular whole milk should not be introduced until your baby is nine to twelve months old and is eating a variety of foods containing iron and vitamin C. It is unsafe to use 2% or skim milk in the first year of life because whole milk is needed for energy and growth.

Giving your baby solid foods

The baby needs breast milk or formula at least four times a day until he is five months old. As he matures, he is able to use his tongue to move food from the front of his mouth to the back, and to swallow and properly digest foods that are not liquids. Bigger babies who are growing quickly may need to start solids at about four months. Other babies can wait until they are about six months.

Your doctor or nurse will help you decide when to start solids.

You can experiment to see if your baby likes it best to have his solids before his milk or after it. Some babies like their solid foods in the middle of a feeding.

What should I give him first?

Start with infant cereals; after a few weeks add vegetable purees, one at time; next add fruit purees. When your baby has had enough time to get used to fruits, it is time to add meat and alternatives. By this time your baby will be around seven or eight months old.

Iron-fortified infant cereals: Until your baby is eighteen months old, this will be his most important type of food after breast milk or formula. Although he was born with a supply of iron in his body, that supply is slowly used up as he grows.

Mix the cereal with some formula, breast milk or water. Some cereals already have dry formula in them, so you just need to add water. Check the label to be sure. Start with about a teaspoon of dry cereal. Make it thin, but give it to the baby with a spoon, not in a bottle.

Give him the same cereal every day for a week. Watch for any rash or upset stomach. When you are sure he can tolerate that cereal, it is time to give him a different kind for a week. Don't give him a mixed cereal until you are sure he can handle each grain in the mix by itself.

Vegetable purees: Give him vegetable purees for a few weeks before you give him fruit purees. If you give fruit first, he may not like the vegetables. Again, try one food at a time for a few days. If it seems to agree with him, try another.

Fruit purees: When he is eating vegetables well, it is time to start on a fruit puree.

Protein purees: Protein purees can be made from meat, fish, poultry, egg yolk, well-cooked legumes, tofu, cottage cheese, cheese or yogurt. Do not add egg white to the diet until after he is a year old.

Fruit juice: Give him about two ounces of fruit juice when he is able to drink from a cup; in fact, when he is about ten months old you can use some juice or water to teach him to drink from a cup.

What should the texture of solid foods be?
Four to six months: Food should be semi-liquid, because the baby is not yet able to chew and swallow. Cereal should be very thin, and vegetables should be pureed.

Six to eight months: The baby needs some practice in chewing, whether he has a few teeth or none at all. If you don't get some chewable foods in now, some babies refuse to accept them for many months.

If you make your own baby food, mash most foods very smoothly with a fork, blender or food grinder, gradually mashing less well. Meat is very hard to chew, so you should continue to give pureed meats until after eight months. If you use commercial baby foods, switch to junior foods when the baby is between seven and nine months old.

You can also begin to give the baby some finger foods: bread crusts, dry toast and cooked vegetables.

After eight months: Start to cut foods up very finely instead of mashing them. At first, give him some mashed foods and some cut-up foods, then slowly increase the proportion of cut-up food. Meat can be cut up very finely.

Good finger foods for babies this age are pieces of soft ripe fruit such as banana, pieces of cooked fruit, pieces of meat and poultry, and cheese cubes.

Dangerous foods

The baby may choke on any of the following foods:

- **raw hard fruits and vegetables** such as carrots, celery, apples or apple peels
- **seeded fruit** such as berries and whole grapes or cherries
- **hot dogs, popcorn, nuts, seeds, chips or small round hard or chewy candies**

Adding a new food

Let your baby get used to one food before you give him another. Add a new food about once a week. That will give you time to make sure the baby doesn't have a bad reaction to it. Watch out for upset stomach, rashes or red patches on the skin.

Give him a tiny bit of a new food—just a teaspoon is enough. If there is no bad reaction, you can give more the next time. Don't give the baby mixed foods until he has had each part of the mixture on its own. For example, don't give him mixed peas and carrots until after he has had both peas and carrots separately.

Add a new food when the baby is calm and happy and you are relaxed. If the baby won't eat the new food, take it away. You can try it again a few days or weeks later.

Your baby won't like everything, but he knows what he likes—at least he knows what he likes today. Next week or next month he may change his mind, just like you.

Solid foods: commercial or homemade?
You can use a blender, food processor or grinder to make baby food. This costs less than commercial baby food, but commercial food may be more convenient. You can use both: homemade when you have time and commercial foods when you are busier.

Although they don't contain salt or other additives, some commercial baby foods have added sugar, so read the labels carefully.

How do I make my own baby food?
Wash your hands before making the puree, and make sure the spoons, knives and blender parts

are really clean. It is best to use fresh fruits and vegetables, but you can also use them frozen or tinned.

Wash fresh fruits and vegetables well, then cook until they are very tender, without adding any salt or sugar. If you use something from a tin, rinse excess salt or sugar off before you use it.

When the baby is old enough for meats, you can use fresh cooked fish, meat or poultry, as well as frozen fish. Canned fish has too much salt.

Blend about a cup of food at a time until it is very smooth. Do not add cooking water when you are blending, because some root vegetables may be high in nitrates, and the nitrates will be in the cooking water. Use fresh water instead.

Store the food in the fridge and throw out what you don't use after three days.

Many parents freeze the purees they make. Put them in an ice cube tray, with enough for one meal in each section. Once the cubes are frozen, put the cubes in a plastic bag or container and date. **Do not refreeze.** Once frozen food has thawed out, throw it away if you don't use it.

Feeding a vegetarian baby

Follow the general guidelines above to introduce your baby to solid foods, starting with iron-fortified infant cereals.

If you eat milk products and eggs, you will have greater choices in giving your child a balanced diet. If you are strict vegetarians, by the time he is twelve to twenty-four months old his diet should look something like this:

- 680 g (24 oz.) of soy formula or milk a day
- four to six tablespoons of iron-fortified cereal
- one or two slices of whole-wheat bread
- one-third to one-half cup of cooked pureed vegetables
- two to three tablespoons of peanut butter or tahini
- four to five servings of fruit and vegetables

Serve well-cooked vegetables or tofu as a substitute for meat.

Vitamins and minerals

If you give your baby formula, he doesn't need any vitamin or mineral supplements.

If you breast-feed your baby, he may need some extra vitamins and minerals:

Vitamin D: Some doctors recommend vitamin D for the first six months, especially if your child won't get much sunshine, which the body needs to make vitamin D.

Vitamin B12: If you are a strict vegetarian, there may not be enough vitamin B12 in your breast milk. Talk to your dietitian for help in deciding how to get enough.

Iron: Breast-fed babies don't need extra iron until about six months. Use baby cereal that has added iron.

Fluoride

Fluoride is a mineral that helps prevent tooth decay. If you live in an area where fluoride is not added to the water supply, you should start giving your baby fluoride supplements by the time he is six months old. Follow the directions carefully. Although a little fluoride is good for you, too much can cause spots on the teeth. You can have your well water tested for fluoride.

Making mealtimes easy

If you watch his body language, you will be able to tell when your baby has had enough. He will turn his head away or lean back in the chair.

Your baby will like some foods and refuse other foods. Some babies are hungrier than others; some find it hard to get used to new foods, and every day is different.

One day your baby will grab the spoon away from you because he wants to feed himself. This is the beginning of a messy and exciting process. Get him a big bib. Cover the floor around his chair. Let him go to it.

Even after he starts to feed himself, he may want you to feed him when he is sick or too excited.

Here are some suggestions for making mealtimes happy:

- Put the food on the baby's tray. Don't give him too much of any one thing. Let him sit and eat with the rest of the family, but don't pay much attention to what he eats or doesn't eat. Talk, relax and enjoy your meal.
- After twenty minutes or so, the meal is over. Take away all the food on your baby's tray. Babies never starve by refusing to eat.

- If you are worried that he doesn't eat enough, make sure he is hungry at mealtime. Give him water instead of juice in the afternoon, and give him a sugarless snack such as a piece of cooked carrot, unsalted cracker or melba toast instead of teething biscuits. When it is mealtime he will be ready to eat most of what you give him.

Chapter 14

Your Baby's First Year

During the first year, your baby will develop a personality of her own; as well as growing bigger, she will learn to use her arms, her legs and her five senses to take control of her environment, and she will learn a lot about getting along with people.

During her first month, take her to a well-baby clinic or to the doctor, and make regular visits after that.

The visiting nurse
In many places, the public health nurse will come to visit you and your baby at home. Call your health unit to ask for a visit from the nurse. You can make the arrangements before the baby is born, at the hospital or when you come home.

Growing bigger
Sometimes she will have a spurt of growth, and at other times she will make slower but steady progress. It doesn't really matter how much the baby grows or how fast. The important thing is that she keeps growing and gaining weight.

At six months she will probably double her birth weight; by the time she is a year old, she

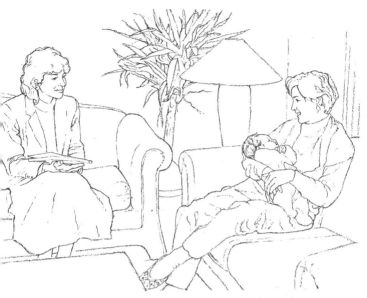

will probably weigh three times as much as she weighed when she was born.

Getting bigger is only one sign of a healthy baby. She should also eat well, sleep well, play actively and learn to do things that are appropriate to her age.

If your baby is getting bigger and learning to do new things, she is all right. You will probably know other babies who may be faster at some things than your baby, and slower at others. Growing up is not a race. You can be happy with the way your baby is developing because she is unique.

Clothing

Most babies wear nightgowns or sleepers. She won't need many other clothes. When she starts crawling, she can wear rompers or overalls. She will need some sweaters, hats and socks.

Clothes for outside

In the summer, the baby can wear rompers, overalls or playsuits. When she is outside, she should wear a hat at all times. A hat will keep her eyes and her head safe from the sun. It is easy for a baby to get too hot. If she sleeps in her carriage, check it often to make sure it is not too hot inside. A baby will get a sunburn very quickly, so don't let her stay in the sun. Ask your doctor about using a sun block cream on her skin when she is outside.

In the winter, don't keep your baby outside too long. To prevent frostbite, make sure her head, hands and feet are well covered. A scarf or a blanket around your baby's face will protect her from the wind, but make sure she can breathe easily.

Clothes for inside

Inside the house, your baby should wear about the same number of clothes you do. If she is sleeping, give her an extra blanket.

Sleeping

Your baby will probably sleep a lot when you first get her home. As she gets older, she will start sleeping in a regular pattern. Feeding her at the same time every day will help her get into the habit of going to sleep at the same time. Some babies are slow to settle into a routine, but a pattern will be established. Once you know when she will be asleep and when she will be awake, you can plan your activities to fit her schedule.

If your baby sleeps through the night, great. However, it is no measure of your worth as a parent, or of your baby's development or intelligence.

At first, the baby will wake up when she is hungry and go to sleep soon after she is fed. Soon she will stay awake for a longer time, wanting to be sociable. Usually babies start with a little play time late in the afternoon; later they make another play time in the morning.

At about six months old, babies usually will sleep for about twelve hours at night, and another three to five hours during the day. By the time they are a year old, they usually take two short naps during the day and sleep a good twelve hours at night.

However, your baby is the best judge of how much sleep she needs. Give her a quiet, warm bedroom, and let her decide how much to sleep. If she doesn't sleep very much and is cranky, or if she seems to be sleepy most of the time, talk to your doctor.

There are many ways to settle a baby down to sleep, but they all involve a quiet time before you put her to bed. Talk to her, cuddle her or sing to her; this will naturally grow into story time as she gets older. After you put her to bed she may talk to herself and wriggle a little before she goes to sleep.

A baby should never be given medicine to make her sleep.

Play time

As the baby stays awake longer, there is more time for play and learning, which are really the same thing for a baby.

When she hears you talk to her, she is learning to understand language. The more you talk to her, the better she will be able to speak later on.

When the baby plays with people, she learns how to get along with others. If they don't tease her or harm her, she learns to like people and to trust them.

Playing with toys helps the baby learn about her body and what she can do. For the first few months, hang some brightly coloured things over her crib to give her something to look at.

When she is three months old, she will be reaching out for everything. If she has a playpen, she will be safe. She can reach out for things and pick them up, and she can go outside in her playpen for some fresh air.

When she is about six months old she will like to watch things as they go by. She will be endlessly entertained by a ride in her carriage or stroller.

Exercise

Even a baby needs exercise. Give her lots of opportunity to move around as much as she can. Let her play with things she has to reach for before she can crawl; then let her chase a big ball. Her muscles will get stronger, and she will also improve her coordination and learn about her own body in relation to the world.

Toys

Whether you buy toys or make them yourself, two questions are important. Are they safe? Are they right for the baby's age?

The first thing to check is the size. The baby will swallow anything she can put in her mouth, so make sure her toys are too big to fit.

Toys should be all in one piece, without little parts that could come off and be swallowed. Check the eyes on stuffed toys.

Toys should be smooth and soft. If they have a sharp edge, the baby will poke herself with it.

Your baby will suck and lick every toy you give her. Make sure the stuffing and the paint or coating are safe if the baby swallows some, and keep them clean.

Your baby needs only a few toys at a time.

Soothers

If you decide to use a soother, buy more than one of the same kind, because babies don't like to change from one kind to another. Make sure it is safe:

- Use an orthodontic soother. These are

specially shaped for the baby's mouth and may prevent dental problems in the future.

- The soother should be strong and easy to clean, and all one piece.
- The plastic guard that keeps the nipple from going too far into the mouth should be too big to fit into the mouth. The guard prevents the baby from swallowing or choking on the soother.
- If there is a cord on the soother, it should be too short to go around the baby's neck.
- Make sure the material is safe for a baby to chew on.
- Don't put sugar, honey or anything sweet on the nipple because they cause tooth decay.
- Wash the soother with warm soapy water and rinse it well.
- When the rubber is worn out, or seems to be sticky, throw it away.
- Buy a new soother before the baby has chewed through her old one.

Sucking the thumb

Some babies need to suck more than others. Many babies suck their thumbs in their mother's uterus.

If the baby sucks her thumb long and hard, until she is two or three years old, the thumb may push the gums and teeth so they stick out. If you are concerned about thumb sucking and tooth formation, see your doctor. A soother may help reduce thumb sucking. Orthodontic soothers, especially designed to fit the shape of the mouth, are recommended.

Dental health

Two things are important for the baby's teeth. The first is good nutrition. The second is keeping sweet and sugary things out of her mouth.

Both the baby teeth and the permanent teeth started to grow in the jaw before the baby was born. To make sure both sets of teeth are healthy, you and the baby must eat well.

Germs in the baby's mouth work on sweet things to produce an acid that makes holes in the teeth. Less acid will be formed if you don't give her fruit drinks or too much juice, and if you clean her teeth. You can use a cloth or a soft brush to clean the baby's teeth as soon as they grow in.

Nursing bottle syndrome

Dentists see young children whose upper front teeth have many cavities; these are caused by the child sleeping with a bottle in her mouth.

Milk, juice or any sweet liquid will stay in the baby's mouth for a long time if she sucks it as she is going to sleep. The acid that forms will have all night to work on her teeth, because there is less saliva in the mouth to wash the acid away. The acid may make holes in her teeth.

Dental problems

Well-cared-for baby teeth prevent many problems with later teeth. For example, if a baby tooth is lost too early, the other baby teeth nearby will move into the space left behind. The permanent tooth may come in crooked if the space is not big enough.

Some babies are born with teeth already showing. Sometimes these are baby teeth and they need to be taken care of as mentioned above. Sometimes they are extra teeth. Your dentist can tell you what to do to take care of them.

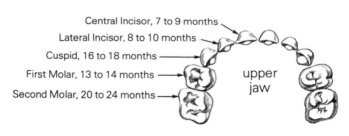

Central Incisor, 7 to 9 months
Lateral Incisor, 8 to 10 months
Cuspid, 16 to 18 months
First Molar, 13 to 14 months
Second Molar, 20 to 24 months

upper jaw

back of mouth

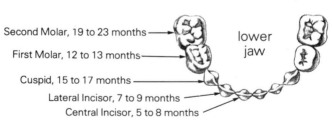

Second Molar, 19 to 23 months
First Molar, 12 to 13 months
Cuspid, 15 to 17 months
Lateral Incisor, 7 to 9 months
Central Incisor, 5 to 8 months

lower jaw

Teething

Usually babies get their first teeth when they are between six and twelve months old. Most babies get the two bottom front teeth first, then the top two teeth. The chart shows the names of the teeth

160

and when you can expect your baby to get hers.

Your baby will have all twenty of her baby teeth by the time she is about two and a half years old.

The most frequent sign of a new tooth is drooling, which starts a few days before a tooth comes in. A bib will help keep the baby's clothes dry.

Babies react to teething differently. She may be a little fussy because her gums are sore.

You can rub her gums with your finger to relieve the soreness, or she may want to chew on a teething ring made of hard rubber or plastic. Even though she has no teeth, chewing will help make her gums hard and exercise the muscles in her jaw.

When she is teething, your baby will chew on anything that she can get in her mouth. Don't let her chew anything made out of wood, because she may swallow slivers. Except for toys made for babies, don't let her chew on anything that has paint on it.

Immunization

At birth a baby is immune to some common childhood diseases. This immunity comes from the mother, and it gradually disappears during the first several months of life. Fortunately, we have vaccines to prevent a number of diseases that have very serious effects and are sometimes even fatal. These diseases include diphtheria, whooping cough (pertussis), tetanus (lockjaw), polio, mumps, red measles and German measles.

If your baby is sick, you should wait until she is better before she is immunized. Often a child will be fussy and irritable or have a slight fever after immunization. If this reaction lasts for more than a day, call your doctor.

Immunization can be done at your doctor's office or at a community health clinic. The immunization timetable will probably be something like this:

Age	Vaccine	Protects against:
2 months	DPT polio and DPT and OPV	Diphtheria, pertussis (whooping cough), tetanus, poliomyelitis (polio)
4 months	DPT polio or DPT and OPV	Diphtheria, pertussis, tetanus, polio
6 months	DPT polio or DPT	Diphtheria, pertussis, tetanus, polio
12 months	MMR	Measles, mumps, rubella (German measles)
18 months	DPT polio or DPT and OPV	Diphtheria, pertussis, tetanus, polio
	Hib	Invasive hemophilus, influenza infection
4 to 6 years	DPT polio or DPT and OPV	Diphtheria, pertussis, tetanus, polio
14 to 16 years	dT polio or dT	Diphtheria, tetanus, polio

DPT = diphtheria pertussis tetanus vaccine
OPV = oral polio vaccine (Sabin)
Hib = Hemophilus influenza b conjugate vaccine
dT = Diphtheria and Tetanus Toxoid for persons 7 years of age and older

Keep a record of the immunizations as your child has them, and take it with you every time you go to the clinic or the doctor. This is a very important record if you move or change doctors or clinics.

Travelling

Generally, if your baby is healthy, she can travel with you. Many babies seem to like travelling in a car and can adapt to most situations.

Is she safe? This is the most important thing to ask when you travel with your baby. Use car seats, seat belts or life jackets as required, and never leave your baby alone, even for a minute.

By car

Buckle up. It's the law. For more information on car safety, read the section called "How do I keep my child safe in the car?" in Chapter 16.

By plane

Many airlines are now allowing certain kinds of car seats to be used on the plane. As well, some airlines have "sky cots" especially for infants. Ask about them when you make your reservations.

To help your baby adjust to the pressure changes of takeoff and landing, bring her on board a little hungry. Burp her before takeoff if possible, and feed her during takeoff. Swallowing and sucking may prevent an earache. If she is not hungry, give her a soother. Repeat the process on the landing.

Check with your doctor if you are going to be flying and your baby has a cold or an ear infection.

Just for partners

Growing, smiling, teething, creeping, talking, immunizations—so many new things are happening in your baby's life. It may seem overwhelming. You may feel you don't know enough to be able to do what's right. Join the club. Nobody's perfect, but your baby doesn't know that. Get involved. Trust yourself to be able to figure out what is best for your baby, and find out where to go for help if you need it. The more time and energy you put into being a parent, the more you'll get out of it. You'll find it's worth every minute.

Chapter 15

Your Baby Grows

In this first year, your baby will grow emotionally and mentally as well as physically.

How he develops depends on many things. The people who look after him help him grow in a certain way, depending on their family customs and beliefs. The family situation of each child is part of his upbringing and experiences. The oldest child in a family is different from the youngest.

Some babies are always on the go. You can never tell what they are going to do next. Others are very happy just to sit until something interesting comes along. Some seem to feel a lot of pain; others fall down and get up without noticing it. Some pay close attention to what is going on around them; others keep their minds on what they are doing and hardly notice anything else.

Every baby learns at his own pace. Here is a guide to a child's development. Your baby may be faster at some things and slower at others. He may be faster or slower at everything and still be normal.

Your baby will grow at the right speed for him. Notice when he does something new. Laugh with him when he learns to sit up or roll over. Whether he is "early" or "late" in learning these things, he will be surprised and pleased with himself. Comparing him with some other child will prevent you from simply enjoying your child's development, and it may make your baby feel anxious.

First month
Your baby likes to look at everything. He will

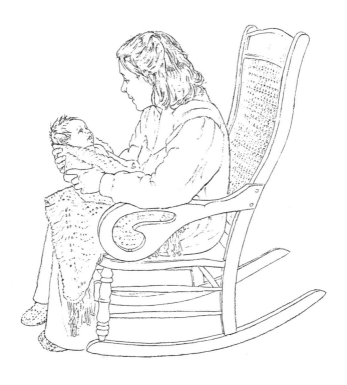

watch your face when you are feeding him, and he may smile when someone smiles at him or plays with him. If you move a light or a toy slowly in front of him, his eyes will follow it along. He likes things with bright patterns more than dull things.

He may laugh and squeal a little, or make soft little noises when he is happy, but most of his sounds will be crying.

He can hear. If you ring a bell, you will see how quiet he gets. If you hold him snugly against your chest, the noise of your heart will quiet him.

He can suck, cry, cough, sneeze and get his hands in his mouth. He may be able to smell things, but not very well.

Soon he will be able to lift his head off the bed when he is lying on his stomach. When lying on his back, he may turn his head to one side or another. Since his neck is not strong enough to hold his head up without help, support his head with your hand when you pick him up.

You may notice some reflexes in the newborn baby.

"Startle" reflex (Moro): When startled, your baby will stretch out his legs and arms, straighten his body, then quickly curl up. By the fourth week this reflex starts to disappear, and it is gone by the end of the sixth month.

Grasp reflex: When you touch the palm of the baby's hand, he will hold onto your fingers and support some or all of his body weight. This reflex disappears by the fifth month.

Rooting reflex: When you touch your baby's

cheek, he will turn his mouth in that direction, open his mouth and look for the nipple. This reflex will not disappear until he stops nursing.

Second month

If you pull his arms to make him sit up, he may be able to hold his head up for a minute or so. Sometime after six weeks and before four months he should be able to hold his head up when he is sitting.

When someone comes towards him, your baby will smile. He likes light and bright colours.

He may start to make a few sounds and may react to music.

If you move a toy in front of him, he will follow it with his eyes all the way from one side of his head to the other side. His eyes should be working well together, and he will no longer be cross-eyed. He learns to hold his hands together in front of him.

Third and fourth months

Sometime in the third or fourth month he will be able to lie on his back and lift his head up for a few minutes. He can't sit up by himself, but when you prop him up he can hold his head up straight. When he is lying on his stomach, he will push himself up on his arms to look around.

He will smile more when someone comes in, especially someone he knows well. He will pull his clothes over his face when he is playing. He will bring his hands together and watch them. He can hold a rattle. If you try to pull a toy out of his hands, he may pull back. He will know his bottle when you show it to him.

When you speak, he will turn towards you. He will coo and laugh and "talk" when he is happy, or when someone talks to him.

Fifth and sixth months

He may start to be afraid of strangers. Up until now, he didn't know some people were strangers and some weren't. If you let him sit where no one will bother him while he watches the stranger, he may get over being afraid.

He is finding his body. He plays with his toes and grabs his feet. He smiles or talks to this face in the mirror. He can hold a rattle easily and can pass a toy from one hand to the other. He will start to reach for toys that are too far away, and he puts everything in his mouth.

He learns to roll over.

He will be able to feed himself a crust of bread. He pats the bottle with both hands when you feed him.

If you make noises at him, he will laugh, chuckle, squeal and make all sorts of sounds; soon he will be saying words.

At about six months he will be able to sit in a highchair; usually he will be able to sit by himself before he is eight months old. If you hold him so he is standing, he will start to put some of his weight on his feet.

Seventh and eighth months

The baby knows his name. He feeds himself a piece of bread or a cracker and holds a bottle. He may start playing peek-a-boo and pat-a-cake, although this may not happen until he is a year old.

He can say four or more different sounds, and he will babble more than ever. He will say "mama" and "dada" before ten months.

He likes to play with paper. He holds things in one hand instead of two. He may hold two toys at once.

Some babies stand up holding onto something. Others start walking around holding onto the chairs or sofas.

Ninth and tenth months

The baby will clap his hands and wave good-bye when you do.

If he is shy or afraid of strangers, he will hang onto people he knows. He may cry if his parents leave.

He is making more sounds than ever. He will shout to get your attention. His sounds start to have meaning.

He may start drinking from a training cup or a regular cup sometime between nine and sixteen months of age. He pokes at things with his finger and will put things into a box and take them out. He will play with a ball on the floor.

He can sit up for as long as he likes. He can pull himself up to stand, holding onto the furniture. He may stand alone for a few moments.

He crawls all over.

He starts to focus on very small things.

Eleventh to fourteenth months

He eats food with his fingers and takes an interest in pictures.

He can hold his arms and legs out. He may start "helping" you dress him. He will give you a toy if you ask for it, and he will try to feed himself with a spoon.

He will be trying to talk all the time, and he may know the meaning of a few words. He will understand things such as "Give me the ball" or "No, no."

He throws toys on the floor on purpose and points to things he wants. If you show him how to pile two blocks up, he will try to do it himself.

He may still be crawling or may walk holding on with two hands, even with one hand. Some babies stand alone well and have started to walk by themselves.

Does my child have a problem?

If your child is slow in one area, it does not mean that he has a problem. If he is very different from the chart, or if he is late in lots of things, you should ask some questions: Has he had the chance to grow and learn? Is there a problem with his health? For example, if he does not respond normally to sounds, it may be because he can't hear well.

Is he eating right? Is there anything else

strange about the things he does? Talk to the child's doctor or the public health nurse. They will be able to answer your questions about the best way to help your baby grow and learn.

How can I help my baby learn?
Babies learn best when they feel safe and secure, and they learn by example.

He wants to learn about the world. You can help him by giving him safe things to touch. He will learn to notice the difference between hard things and soft things, wet and dry, rough and smooth, round and square.

Give him lots of different things to hear; make faces at him, and let him copy you; roll around on the floor or bed with your baby.

He wants to learn how to do things. Give him the chance to try to do new things. If he knows you have confidence in him, he will try something new, and try it again and again until he gets it. Notice his efforts. Tell him he is a smart kid.

Enjoy your baby. Help your whole family to enjoy him. Everybody in the family can learn along with your baby.

Play
Play is important to your baby's development. Through play a child learns new skills, gains confidence, learns how to get along with others, and expresses his feelings.

Babies need some time by themselves. They can play by themselves for a while, especially if they know you're not too far away.

Discipline

A child needs to learn to behave so he can get along with other people. He needs to know that he can't please only himself but has to cooperate with others. Your baby will copy the examples he sees around him. His parents are the most important people in his life, and he will try to be just like you.

When your baby starts moving around, he will get into places that are not safe. Act quickly. Give him something else to play with, or pick him up and take him somewhere safe. Tell him why you are doing it.

Eventually you will have to teach him the meaning of "no" to keep him safe. Save the "no" for times when there is real danger—like a hot stove.

Don't spank him. If you spank him, he learns to be afraid of you. He learns it's okay for a big person to hit a little person. When he gets a chance, he will hit smaller children, and he will hit you.

Instead of spanking him, watch for him to do something you like. Give him a hug or a smile to tell him you approve. He wants your attention, so reward him when he does something you like. He'll want to do that again.

If he's doing something you don't like, give him something else to do. This works best with younger children.

If he's drawing on the wall, give him some

paper to draw on.

If he's being too rough in the living room, take him outside to play, or into his bedroom.

It is better to make the house safe for him than to keep saying "no!"

Setting rules

Set clear rules about behaviour, and enforce them. Make as few rules as possible, but be consistent with them. If you don't let children play noisy games in the living room, stop them every time. If your children know what the rules are, they will start disciplining themselves.

Be sure your child is old enough to understand the rule. Explain the rules often. Let other adults know what the rules are.

How to enforce the rules? Call time out. Simply removing a child from a situation is usually enough to stop the behaviour. A quiet time will give him some time to cool off after a rule has been broken. Three to five minutes is enough.

Sometimes I get so mad!

Sometimes parents get angry. Try to let your child know that you still love him, even though you are angry at his behaviour.

If you do lose your temper, say you're sorry when you calm down. An apology will make you both feel better, and it sets a good example for your child. If he never sees anyone apologize, how can he learn how to do it himself?

What should I do if I think I might hurt my child?

When you feel anger building up inside you, and you are afraid you will hurt your child, leave the room. It is better to leave the child alone for a few minutes than to risk hurting him.

Find a way to let off steam that won't hurt anyone. Run, jump, shout, hit a pillow, throw ice cubes in the bathtub. Everyone feels angry or frustrated sometimes. What matters is how you show your anger.

Call a friend, a family member, a help line, a hospital emergency room, Parents Anonymous, or anyone you trust who can help you or who might know where to get help.

Help yourself before you hurt your child.

Make time for your baby

As he gets older, your baby will want to play all the time. When you are feeding him, or bathing him, or getting him dressed, he will want to play. Since he learns when he plays, try not to rush him. Enjoy your baby and the time you spend with him.

Housework can always wait, and some things will have to slide. No one will notice the dust on the baseboards, for example, but the toys all over the floor are dangerous, and the mess will make you frantic. Take a few minutes to pick up the toys, and forget about the baseboards.

Will something terrible happen if I don't do this job? If the answer is yes, do the job. If the answer is no, spend time having fun with your family.

Often a baby will be happy just to be in the same room with you while you work, where he can watch you move around and you can talk to him. This soon develops into the baby "helping" you—another of the joys of having a child in your life.

Fears

Fear helps a baby stay out of trouble. He will be afraid of loud or sudden noises, falling, moving too fast and so on. Children learn to be afraid in certain situations. For example, if a big dog scares them, they may be afraid of all dogs. They will be afraid if they can sense that someone around them is afraid.

Try to prepare him for things that might scare him. He will be less fearful if you let him know in advance when you are going to make a loud noise, or when the car is coming up to a dark tunnel.

When he is scared, take his fears seriously. Don't make fun of him for being afraid. Instead, let him know that he is safe with you. Don't make him do something that he is afraid to do. If he is afraid of the dark, leave a light on.

If a fear gets out of hand and seems to be taking over a large part of your child's life, ask your doctor or mental health worker for advice.

Older children

It takes time for children to get used to a new

baby. They may be jealous of the time you spend with the new little one, especially if you seem too busy for them. When people bring presents and make a fuss over the new baby, it doesn't seem fair. Children can think that no one loves them. They may get very upset.

You can tell your older child you understand that it's hard to get used to a new baby.

- Make sure she can't harm the new baby.
- Give her a chance to tell you how she feels, without trying to judge her feelings or change them.
- If your older child acts like a baby, let her be a baby. Cuddle her and take care of her until she feels safer and more loved.
- Praise her, encourage her, and make her feel good about herself and her accomplishments.
- Make a special time for you and your older child every day.

Grandparents and other relatives
Grandparents, aunts, uncles and other family members may have lots to give to your baby. Your baby will be glad to find other adults who love him and will play with him, or read or talk to him. You will enjoy having a break from your baby while someone else is caring for him, and he is getting to know the rest of the family.

Sitters
You will need someone to look after the baby from time to time. If you have a family member

who can do it, so much the better. If you have a friend or a neighbour with children, you can take turns looking after each other's children while the parents go out. However, there will probably be times when you have to find a sitter outside your immediate circle of friends and family. Finding a sitter you feel comfortable with will be one of your biggest challenges. Ask other parents in your neighbourhood. Try to find someone who has taken a course in babysitting or who has some experience.

It is a good idea to invite the sitter over to visit before you go out and leave the baby. The baby can meet the sitter and you can show her or him around your home.

When you go out, the sitter needs to know where the baby sleeps, where you keep the food and clothing and how to lock up the house. It may be a good idea to leave written instructions about how to feed the baby and how to calm him if he cries.

Be sure to leave some emergency numbers near your phone. Include a number where you can be reached, a neighbour's number and your complete address, in case the sitter has to call the fire department or an ambulance and tell them where to come.

Day care while you work

If you are going back to work, you will need someone to look after your child every day. You could put your child in a day-care centre, or in a day-care home; a family member could look after him or you could have a nanny come into your home.

Seventy per cent of women with young children go out to work or to school daily. Like them, you may feel worried or guilty about leaving your child with a caregiver. Certainly you may miss holding and playing with your child for many hours every day. However, you can be sure that your child will do well in a safe, warm and stimulating place.

Even though a child spends many hours a day at day care, his parents will remain the most important people in his life. Your love and your values will mean more to him than those of his caregivers.

How will my child adjust to going to day care?
If you are positive about the fun he will have, and if you seem to like and trust the caregivers, he will follow your lead.

However, it is not easy for a child to change his routine. You can expect that he may go back to a less mature stage for a few days or a couple of weeks. He may want to cuddle more when at home, or be more fussy, or insist you feed him instead of wanting to feed himself. He needs to feel secure in your love. Give him what he needs; he will return quickly to his old habits.

Long before you are ready to send him to day care, make sure he has a chance to be around many different adults. Let others cuddle him or change him or play with him while you are near. If he is used to several caregivers, he will not find it so hard to go to day care.

What kind of day care is available?
Start looking at your options long before you go back to work. You will need time to search out what is available in your area, and time to visit day-care centres and day-care homes, check on references, apply for subsidies if you are eligible and so on. As well, many day-care centres have waiting lists of up to a year. Here are some options to think about:

Unlicenced home day care: This is an informal arrangement for day care in a private home, usually that of a family member or a neighbour.

Licenced home day care: Caregivers are supervised in their homes by a licenced agency or by government agencies.

Group day-care centre: Larger groups of children are cared for in a licenced space designed especially for children.

Nanny: You may hire a nanny to live in your home or to come in daily to look after your child.

How do I choose?
Go and visit day-care homes and centres in your area. You will find centres listed in the yellow pages of the phone book; for home day care, you may find a list at the community centre, health unit or social services office, or see an ad in the newspaper.

When you visit, ask questions about safety, health, snacks and meals, activities for children and so on. Look around. Do the children there seem happy and safe? Do children get individual time with the caregivers? Will your child get enough fresh air and exercise? What kind of discipline does the caregiver give? What are the rules for behaviour? Do the caregivers seem interested in children? Are they happy with their work?

You are looking for a place that is safe and stimulating, and one that has the same kind of rules and discipline that you use at home.

Ask for references, and check them out.

Contracts

Make sure you have an clear agreement about what you will pay, when you will pay, how much extra you will pay if you are late picking your child up, and if you will have to pay for days your child doesn't go to day care because of illness or other reasons.

Find out about the policy on illness. How sick is too sick for the child to come to day care? In the case of a day-care home, does the caregiver have a backup for when she is sick? You might also interview that person.

Subsidies

Day care is expensive, especially infant care. Day-care centres are generally more expensive than home-care arrangements, while having a nanny can be the most expensive of all.

There are some subsidies available at day-care centres. If you get a subsidy, you will pay only part of the fee; the other part will be paid by the local, provincial and federal governments. However, in most parts of the country there are two-year waiting lists for subsidized infant care. Apply early. To find out how to apply, call your provincial social services, community services or health department.

Just for partners

Enjoy your baby's growth and development. Find time to spend with him and have fun. Looking after him when he is sick, hurt or unhappy may make you feel especially close.

As you begin to understand what parenthood involves, you and your partner will have many things to share—feelings, hopes and fears. Talking to each other about them will build a stronger parenting partnership.

There are many decisions to make about diet, toys, day care, doctors and so on. These are decisions for the partnership to make, so get involved in the research. Visit day-care homes or call to check on references; go to the doctor with the family; do some reading or ask some questions.

Share the work of looking after the baby. When you and your partner are dividing up the jobs, you may find that choosing to stay home to do housework instead of going to buy groceries is your best bet. You get to spend some time with the baby—and folding the laundry with an ten-month-old to help you can be quite an experience. Your partner gets to go outside and shop by herself. Even buying groceries can be a thrill to someone who has been home with a baby for a while.

Find someone who can look after the baby so you can both get out together. Regular time off is good for parents and for their children.

Chapter 16

Safety and First Aid

Don't let injuries happen!

Your child learns by looking and touching and moving around. She is interested in everything. It's up to you to keep her safe.

Every week your child can do something new. As she grows, try to keep one step ahead of her in your mind so you can make your house safe for every stage.

Before she learns to crawl, think about the dangers in your house: a crawling baby could fall down stairs, open low cupboards, grab electrical cords, and pull on tablecloths and anything else that hangs down.

Before she learns to walk, think about the dangers in your house: a walking baby can reach up to the top of the stove, get up on top of things and fall off, get into higher cupboards and so on. A baby this age has more strength to open bottles or containers and will eat or drink what is inside.

Keep thinking ahead as your baby grows. Get down on the floor, where you can see from her point of view, and remove anything that might cause an injury.

- Never leave your baby alone in the house, not even for a minute while you run next door. It doesn't matter if she is asleep or awake. Injuries happen very quickly.

- Never leave your baby alone in the bath, or lying on a table, or playing on the floor, or in a baby seat on a table or counter, or in a highchair, or on a couch or bed.
- Never leave your baby alone with a toddler, a jealous older child or a jealous pet.
- Never leave your infant alone with a propped bottle, since she may choke. She should always be held when being fed.

When do injuries happen?
Children are most often injured at certain times of the day, and at certain times of the year:
- **Early in the morning** when everyone is rushing around, cooking breakfast and getting ready for school or work, or when children are up and parents are still in bed.
- **Right around supper time**, between 5:00 and 7:00 P.M., when you're busy getting supper and family members may be tired.
- **During the summer** when kids are outside and it's harder to keep an eye on them.
- **When there is a change in the family routine:** when someone is visiting, when parents are worried about something else, when someone is sick, when you are moving, when you have lost a job or when parents are fighting.

Why do injuries happen?
There are many causes of injuries; often two or three things combine to cause one.

- Children need to touch things and explore.
- Children grow and change so fast. Today they can do something they couldn't do yesterday. It's hard for parents to keep up with them.
- Children don't know what is not safe. Everything seems fun to them; they don't think about danger.

Be prepared

1. Write down all the phone numbers you might need in an emergency. Put them on the wall near your phone.

- **911.** If you have the 911 system in your area, you can call 911 in any emergency. The operator will ask for your address and will want to know what is happening; he or she will call for whatever kind of help you need.

   If you don't have the 911 system in your area, write down the numbers to call if you need the police, the fire department, the ambulance or the poison control centre.
- your doctor
- two taxi companies
- a crisis line or distress centre
- numbers for two friends or relatives, at home and at work

2. Get a first-aid kit ready, including the following items:

- absorbent cotton
- cotton-tipped swabs
- soap for cleaning cuts
- sterile gauze pads

186

- bandages, 2.5 cm (1 in.) and 5 cm (2 in.)
- adhesive tape 2.5 cm (1 in.)
- tube of antibacterial cream, 30 g (1 oz.)
- scissors
- tweezers
- band-aids
- syrup of ipecac, which will cause vomiting
- a large square of cloth
- calamine lotion

3. Learn infant and child C.P.R. (cardiopulmonary resuscitation) and what to do in case of choking.

Classes are often held to teach these two first-aid measures. For more information, call your public health unit, community college or school board.

What kinds of injuries are most common for kids?
Children are killed or injured most often by:
- car accidents
- fires
- drowning
- falls
- burns
- poisoning

How do I keep my child safe in the car?
Car accidents kill and injure more children than anything else. Your child is forty or fifty times more likely to die in a car accident than from any disease she might catch.

Buckle up. It's the law.

Put your baby in an approved car seat to bring her home from the hospital, and make sure she is safely buckled in every time she gets in a car. You cannot hold onto the baby in a car accident. If there is an accident, the baby will fly out of your arms and be harmed.

You must put the seat in the car the right way. Be sure to follow the directions. You must fasten the safety straps correctly. If you don't use the seat correctly, it cannot prevent an injury.

Choose the right seat for your child

For a child who weighs up to 9 kg (20 lb.), the only safe way to travel in a car is in an infant seat

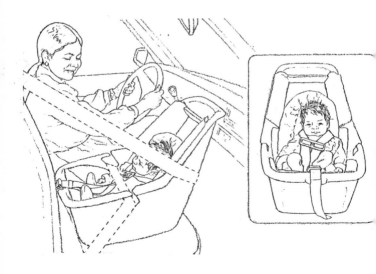

that faces the back of the car.

A child who weighs between 9 and 18 kg (20 to 40 lb.) will need a child car seat. It should face forward in the back seat and be fastened with an adult seat belt. Be sure it meets current safety standards and has been properly installed.

If you are borrowing or renting a car seat, be sure to get one that has never been in an accident. If it has been in one accident, it may not stand up to another.

Many groups offer to lend or rent car seats for children: nurses' groups, hospitals, the Red Cross, service clubs and others. It is usually cheaper to rent or borrow one than to buy it.

Most accidents happen close to home. Buckle up every time, even if you aren't going very far.

General car safety
- Don't let a child stand or kneel on any seat while the car is moving.
- Never leave your baby or small child alone in a car.
- Take the cigarette lighters out of your car. Make sure you look for lighters in the back seat, too.
- Your car should have locks on the back doors that your child can't unlock.
- Always apply the parking brake to prevent the car from rolling.

Safe furniture for children

Playpen

- Slats should be close together so the baby can't get her head caught between them. They should be 6 cm (2.4 in.) apart at most. If you have a mesh playpen, the holes should be very small.
- The playpen should have a strong floor with a foam pad on it.
- The hinges should hold well and not pinch.
- Sides should be 122 cm (48 in.) high.
- It should have no more than two castors or wheels on it.
- Don't string toys across the playpen.
- Keep it away from blinds with long cords.
- Don't use it after the child can climb out of it.

Crib

- Don't use a crib that was made before September 1986. The date should be on the crib. Cribs made before that date are not safe.
- The mattress should fit snugly. Try to put two fingers between the mattress and the side of the crib. If both fingers fit, the mattress is too small.
- Never put a pillow in the crib.

Baby seat

- The bottom should be wide and strong.
- The seat should have a non-slip base.
- Use the safety straps.
- Do not put it on the table. Use it only on the floor.

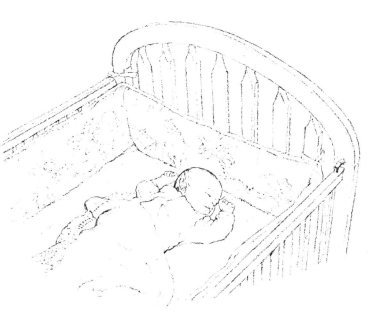

Highchair

- The chair should have a wide base so it is not tippy.
- Use the safety belt or harness all the time.
- Make sure there are no sharp edges on the tray.
- Keep the chair away from the stove.

Walkers

Don't use a walker. They are involved in many cases of injuries to babies, and babies don't need them to learn how to walk.

Making your home safe
Kitchen

- Turn the handles of your pots in towards the back of the stove. Don't let them hang over the front of the stove. Keep the baby away from the oven.
- Keep cleaners, chemicals and poisons up high in a locked cupboard.
- Keep knives and sharp tools out of reach.
- Keep toasters, electric frying pans and other appliances unplugged. Keep them away from water.
- Don't let cords hang down.
- Have a fire extinguisher handy. Make sure it is ready to use.
- When you have finished ironing, put the iron away. Don't leave the ironing board up.
- Keep plastic bags out of reach. Tie knots in thin plastic bags and recycle them. Use paper or cloth bags whenever you can. They are better for the environment, and paper and cloth bags are not dangerous for the baby.
- Keep the garbage can out of reach.

Bathroom

- Make sure no one can slip in the tub. Use non-skid strips or mats.
- Never leave the baby alone in a bath. Always check the temperature of the water before you put the baby in it.
- Keep hair dryers, shavers and anything else that runs on electricity out of the bathroom.

- Keep drugs, cleaners, shampoo, deodorant, hair spray and razor blades up high in a locked cupboard.
- Leave the toilet lid down.

Living room
- Keep plants out of reach. Check to see if the leaves or seeds of any of your plants are poisonous and give those away. Some common poisonous plants are: castor-bean (seeds), dieffenbachia, caladium, some philodendrons, elephant's ears, hyacinth, narcissus and daffodil bulbs, rosary-pea (seeds), holly (berries), Jerusalem cherries, mistletoe (berries) and poinsettias.
- Put a screen in front of fireplaces.
- Don't hang clothes, paper or books near the fireplace or wood stove.
- Don't drink hot beverages or smoke while the baby is in your arms or on your lap.
- Put away lamps, pictures, vases and anything else that could be pulled off tables.
- Remember that your child will try to climb anything—stools, furniture, stepladders, even large toys.

Bedroom
- Keep the crib or playpen away from blinds with long cords and away from dressers with things that can be pulled off the top.
- Use only cold-water humidifiers, never hot-water vaporizers.

- Babies can't move away from things that might smother them. A firm, flat surface is the safest place for a baby. A waterbed is too soft.

Halls and stairs
- Do not use mats or small rugs.
- Use a gate at the top and bottom of the stairs.
- Make sure the stairs are well lit, and keep them clear.
- Leave a light on at night in the hall from the bedrooms to the bathroom.
- Install smoke detectors throughout the house according to fire regulations.

Basement and storage rooms
- Take the doors off fridges, freezers and all appliances that you are not using.
- Turn the water heater down. It should be 50° C (122° F) at most. Ask the power company or an electrician how to turn it down if you are not sure what to do.
- If you have a wringer washer, make sure the safety release on the wringer is working. Unplug it when you are not using it, or when you are using it and you have to go away for a minute.
- Keep paint, paint removers, insecticides and poisons locked up in a high cupboard.
- Keep tools out of reach or locked up. Unplug power tools when you aren't using them.
- Never store gasoline, garden sprays or any other chemicals in pop bottles.

- Keep your child away from dangerous appliances such as lawn mowers, washers, dryers, woodworking tools and machinery.

Pets

Be sure your pets have rabies and distemper shots.

Don't leave pet food sitting out where the baby can eat it.

Never leave a baby alone with a jealous pet. If your pet is jealous, try to make him more secure and help him accept the baby. If you can't get him to accept the baby, find him another home or turn him into an outside pet.

Cats and dogs can spread worms to your baby. Have your pets checked regularly by your vet to make sure they are not infected.

Other things to remember

- Cover electrical outlets with safety caps or heavy tape.
- Tape electrical cords to the wall.
- Unplug outside electrical extension cords when not in use.
- Plan your escape route out of the house in case of fire. Plan another way out in case your first route is blocked by smoke or flames.
- Put safety gratings or strong screens on all upstairs windows. Be sure you can open them if there is a fire.
- If you have big glass doors, put tape or stickers on them so people will see them and not try to walk through them.

- Keep guns unloaded and locked away.
- Keep ammunition locked away in another place. Don't keep guns and ammunition in the same place.
- Pick up all small things a baby could put in her mouth. Put them away where she can't reach them. Some examples are buttons, coins, hard candies, nuts, earrings, cigarettes and cigarette butts.
- Keep outside doors and balcony doors locked at all times.
- Lock all windows; don't rely on screens to keep a child safe.
- Tie blind and drapery cords out of reach.

Outdoor safety

Don't let children play in a driveway.

Be careful in parking lots—hang onto your child's hand, because other drivers can't see her behind a parked car.

If you make sure children always wear shoes outside, they will avoid many cuts, scrapes, puncture wounds and infections.

Your yard should be fenced, with a locked gate.

When children are outside, they should always be supervised, even if they are taking a nap.

Be sure playground equipment is safe.

Water is very dangerous; never leave a child alone in a wading pool, near a swimming pool, on the beach or near an open ditch or a pond. Teach your child to swim as early as possible.

Boating safety

Everyone in the boat should wear a life jacket all the time, including babies and adults who can swim.

Boats must have:
- **life jackets for each person**
- a bailing bucket or pump
- two oars and oarlocks, or two paddles
- a fire extinguisher
- a whistle or horn
- a flotation cushion or a floating line to throw to someone in the water
- six distress flares
- lights on the top and front of the boat

Make sure the boat is securely tied up to the dock. Keep children away from the motor.

Farm safety

Keep children away from fields at harvest time, and keep them away from machinery and tools any time. Don't let them ride on tractors and other large machines.

Lock up fertilizers, chemicals and pesticides.

Keep small children away from large animals.

If you are working in the barn, do not leave the baby alone in the house. Provide a safe place, like a playpen, for her in the barn.

Snowmobile safety

Children under five should never be on a snowmobile, except in an emergency. If you and your children must travel by snowmobile, make sure

that:
- you both wear helmets, face masks, woollen hats and two pairs of mittens
- you travel on well-marked trails
- you tell someone where you are going and when you'll be back
- you never travel at night
- you watch out for fences, posts and clotheslines
- you stay off roads and railroad tracks
- you stay off ice
- you go slowly and check the child often to be sure he's warm and well covered

When to call for help

If you have the 911 system in your area, call 911 for help.

If you can't get your doctor or health care unit on the phone, take the child to the nearest hospital.

Get help if:
- The baby swallows anything other than food.
- The baby chokes on anything and has trouble breathing.
- The baby is scalded by hot water or burned in any other way.
- The baby has an injury to her head.
- The baby is bleeding a lot and it doesn't stop right away.
- You think a bone may be broken or sprained. A small baby's bones don't break as easily as an older child's, but they can bend and splinter. You may not be able to tell for sure.

- The baby has taken something small and pushed it up her nose, into her ears or into her vagina.
- Your child is unconscious.

FIRST AID

Burns

If the baby's clothes are on fire, wrap her in a blanket, coat or rug. This will smother the fire and put it out.

Call for help at once. Do not put anything on the burn.

If the skin is red or has a blister:

1. Put the burned area in cold water for at least two minutes. If the baby is burned by **paint remover, bleach, battery acid, lye, quick lime or another chemical**, rinse the burned part with lots of cool water for at least five minutes.
2. Don't rub the burned area dry. Put the towel over it and press down a very little bit. This will blot up the water.
3. Cover it with a dry, clean towel or non-stick gauze.
4. Lift up the burned part so it is higher than the child's heart. If the burn is on the arm, lift the child's arm up. If it is on the leg, lay the child down with her leg up on a pillow.
5. Do not put butter, creams, ointments or medicine on the burn.
6. If blisters form, do not break them.

Get help for any big burn. Get help for any burn on the face, hands or feet.

Poisons

If you think your child has taken poison, call the poison control centre and follow their instructions.

- Save the jar or can the poison came in, or a bit of whatever the child has eaten.
- If the child vomits, save some of the vomit. The poison control centre may tell you to make the child vomit. You can buy **syrup of ipecac** at the drugstore to make your child vomit. Buy two bottles and keep it out of reach of children. **Don't give it to your child unless the poison control centre tells you to.** Sometimes it is useful to have the child vomit up whatever she has swallowed, but other times it can do more harm. Some poisons burn the throat and mouth. If you make the child vomit, the poison will burn going down and again coming up.

If the baby passes out, do not give her anything to eat or drink. If she passes out, do not try to make her vomit.

Put the number of the poison control centre on your phone or on the wall near your phone if you don't have the 911 system in your area.

Choking (baby)

If the baby can breathe, speak or cough, encourage coughing and stand by to help. Don't

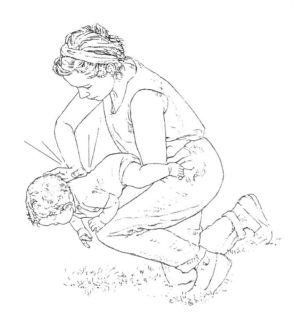

try to pull the object out. Let the baby try to
cough it up on her own. If the baby is turning
blue, can't breathe, can't speak or can't cry, then
you must act quickly.

1. Place the baby face down along your arm. Use
   your hand to support the head and neck.
2. With the heel of your other hand, strike
   sharply between the shoulder blades four
   times.
3. If this doesn't help, turn the baby face up on
   your arm, supporting the head in your hand.
   • Support your arm on your thighs so that the

baby's head is lower than the chest.

- Draw an imaginary line from one of the baby's nipples to the other.
- Put two fingers on the breastbone a little below this imaginary line.
- Press sharply four times.

4. If necessary, repeat blows to the back and thrusts to the chest until the object is out or the baby becomes unconscious.

If the baby becomes unconscious, send for help immediately. Meanwhile, you must try to clear whatever is blocking the airway.

1. Lay the baby face up on a firm, flat surface.
2. Put your thumb into the baby's mouth on top of her tongue and hold her chin with your fingers.
3. Holding onto the tongue and chin, lift upwards.
4. Look into her mouth and use your index finger to pull out anything you see. **Do not poke around. Only try to remove things you can see.**
5. Place your mouth over the baby's mouth and nose, making an airtight seal.
6. Give a gentle puff of air. **If the baby's chest rises,** give a new puff of air every three seconds. Remove your mouth after each puff to let the air out. **If the baby's chest doesn't rise,** repeat blows to the back and thrusts to the chest. Try again to clear the airway and breathe into the baby.

7. Repeat these steps until the baby can breathe alone or medical help arrives.

Some foods that can cause choking are weiners, nuts, popcorn, raw carrots, raw celery and apple skins.

Choking (child)
If the child can breathe, speak or cough, get her to cough and stand by to help. Don't try to pull the thing out. Let the child try to cough it up on her own. If the child is turning blue, can't breathe, can't speak or can't cry, then you must act quickly. Try to get help. Tell someone else to phone 911.
1. Give abdominal thrusts.
   - Get behind the child.
   - Put your arms around the child's waist.

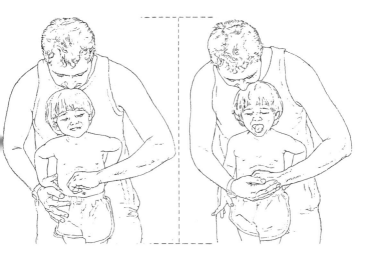

- With one hand, run your finger down the middle of the child's chest until you find the soft spot at the end of the breastbone.
- With your other hand, find the child's bellybutton. Make a fist with your thumb inside. Put your fist just above the bellybutton and well below the soft spot at the end of the breastbone.
- Hold your fist in your other hand.
- Press up, quick and hard.

2. Repeat abdominal thrusts until the object is out. Loosen your hold after you press each time so that each thrust is separate.

If the child passes out, send for help immediately. Meanwhile, you must try to clear whatever is blocking the airway.

1. Lay the child face up on a firm, flat surface.
2. Put your thumb into the child's mouth on top of her tongue and hold her chin with your fingers.
3 Hold onto the tongue and chin and lift up.
4. Look into the mouth and sweep with your index finger to pull out anything you see. **Do not poke around blindly. Only try to remove things you can see.**
5. Pinch the child's nose closed and place your mouth over her mouth, making an airtight seal.
6. Breathe gently into the child's mouth. **If the child's chest rises,** give a new breath of air every four seconds. Remove your mouth after each puff to let the air out. **If the child's chest doesn't rise,** repeat the thrusts to her abdomen.

Try again to clear the airway and to breathe into the child.
7. Repeat these steps until the child can breathe alone or until medical help arrives.

Young children will put almost anything in their mouths. Some foods that can cause choking are weiners, nuts, popcorn, raw carrots, raw celery and apple skins. **Any small thing can cause choking.**

Rescue breathing
In an emergency, don't put yourself in danger. You can't help others if you are injured.

If the child does not seem to be breathing, call for help, then get ready to start rescue breathing:
1. Check for breathing. Put your cheek close to the child's nose and mouth. Watch to see if the chest rises.
2. If the child is not breathing, tip her head back to open the airway. Check for breathing again.
3. If the child isn't breathing, start rescue breathing.

For a baby:
4. Place your mouth over the baby's nose and mouth, making an airtight seal.
5. Give a gentle puff of air.
6. Remove your mouth to let the baby breathe out.
7. Check to make sure the chest rises when you blow air in.
8. Give her a new puff of air every three seconds.

seconds. Remember to remove your mouth after each puff.

9. Keep it up until the baby is breathing again.

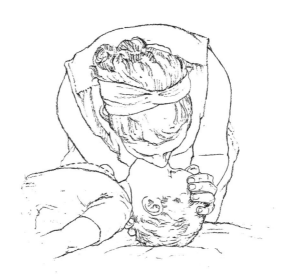

For a child:

4. Pinch nose closed.
5. Cover the child's mouth with yours, making an airtight seal.
6. Breathe gently into the child's mouth.
7. Remove your mouth to let the child breathe out.
8. Check to make sure the chest rises.
9. Give a new breath every four seconds. Remember to remove your mouth after each breath.

10. Keep this up until the child is breathing again. **Get help.**

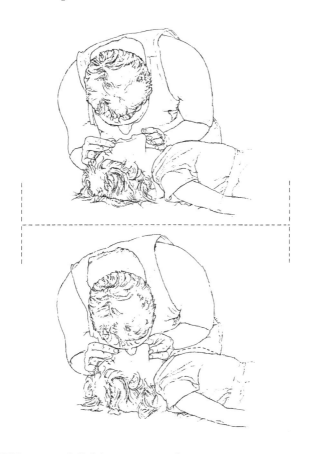

When a child is unconscious
Be sure that the child is breathing and that any bleeding is stopped before you worry about him

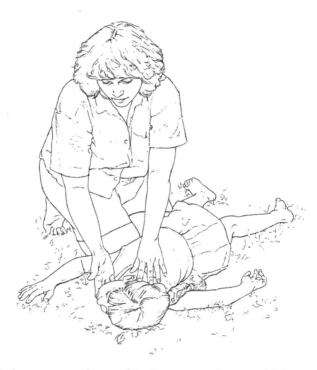

being unconscious. If he is unconscious and lying on his back, he may choke.

1. Kneel beside the child and gently but firmly roll him into the recovery position. To do this:

- Tuck the arm closest to you along the child's side.
- Bring the other arm across the chest.
- Support the head with one of your hands.
- Reach across and hold the waist with your

other hand.

- Roll the child towards you, resting his chest and stomach against your legs.
- Bend the child's top knee towards you so he won't roll forward. Bend the arm closest to you to give him more support.
- Carefully lift the head up and back to help him breathe easily.

If the child is unconscious and lying on his stomach or side, do not move him.

1. Carefully tip the child's head up and back. This will straighten the neck and make breathing easier.
2. Watch carefully to be sure breathing doesn't stop.
3. Loosen any tight clothes.
4. Do not give the child anything to drink.
5. Do not leave an unconscious child alone.

Falls, sprains and fractures

When your baby falls down, take a look at her before you pick her up. If she cries and moves her head and arms and legs, there is probably nothing seriously wrong. Pick her up and comfort her.

If she doesn't move some part of her body, don't move her. If you think a bone is broken, call for help. Don't move the arm or leg that is hurt. Keep the hurt part still. Don't give the child anything to eat or drink.

If you have to move the child, make a splint. A splint is something hard that will help to keep the hurt arm or leg still. Use a board, a stick, a folded newspaper or an umbrella. Put a towel, a shirt or some cloth on top of the hurt part. Then put the splint on. Tie the splint in place. You can use a belt, scarf, tie, rope or string. Don't tie it too tight; make it just tight enough to keep it there without moving.

If you think the neck or back is hurt, do not move the child. **Do not even roll her over.** Try to keep the head from moving. Roll up some towels or blankets. Put one on each side of the head so it can't move. **Get help fast.**

Lumps and bumps on the head
Use cold compresses or an ice pack to reduce swelling and pain.

That night, wake the child every two hours to make sure she's conscious. If the child is unconscious, even for a few seconds, take her to the hospital.

When to get help:

If you notice any of these signs, even after several days, take your child to a hospital:

- unusual sleepiness
- vomiting
- unsteady arms or legs
- slurred words
- a bad headache
- convulsions
- blood or clear liquid coming from ears or nose
- the pupil of one eye is bigger than the other
- the child's eyes don't seem to move together

Cuts and bleeding
Small cuts
- Wash your hands before you look after the cut.
- Wash the hurt part with soap and water. If it is a scrape, clean out the dirt. Use hydrogen peroxide to help clean it.
- Cover a cut with a band-aid or gauze pad. Leave scrapes and scratches uncovered. The air will help them heal.

Get medical help if:
- the cut gets more sore, red or swollen, or if pus comes out of it
- the edges of the cut are spread apart
- you can't get all the dirt out
- the cut is on the lip, eyelid or eyebrow
- something like a fishhook or glass is stuck in the cut

Your child may need a tetanus shot if her shots are not up to date.

Heavy bleeding
If you can't stop the bleeding, make a pile of layers of gauze or paper tissues. Hold it over the spot. Hold it tightly for a few minutes until the blood stops. If the blood comes through the gauze, don't take it off. Put more gauze on top, and press it down. If the bleeding is on an arm or leg, and if you are sure it is not broken, lift it up on a pillow. Put it higher than the heart. This will help stop the bleeding.

After the bleeding slows down, wrap the

bandage firmly around the pad or cloth. Don't make it too tight. You don't want to cut off the circulation. Keep the leg or arm lifted up higher than the heart.

Call your doctor.

Bites and stings
Animal or human bites
If an animal or another person bites your child, check to see if the skin is broken. If it is broken, get medical help. The bite could get infected. Your child might need a tetanus shot.

Wash the bite with soap and water.

Cover it with a gauze pad or clean cloth for the trip to the doctor.

Bee and insect stings
Use tweezers to take out the stinger.

Wash the sting with soap and water. You can put an ice pack or a cold, wet cloth on it. This will take away some of the pain.

Put calamine lotion on it, or mix up some baking soda with a little water and put that on the sting.

If any part of your child's body swells up, get help. She may be allergic to stings. If she has a bad allergy, you might need to get a sting kit. Ask your doctor. He or she can give you a prescription for a sting kit and show you how to use it.

Slivers

Wash the area with soap and water. Use a needle or tweezers to take out the sliver. Use rubbing alcohol to clean the needle or tweezers before you take out the sliver.

If there are many slivers, or if they are deep or dirty, you may want to see your doctor.

Something in the eye

Wash your hands. Try to keep the baby from rubbing her eye. Wrap her snugly in a blanket or towel so she can't move around too much while you are looking after her eye.

If there is a bit of dirt in it, lift up the top lid and bring it down over the bottom lid. Hold it for a moment or two.

You could also wash out the eye with water. It should be lukewarm, not hot and not cold. Use a clean dropper or a clean spoon to drop the water into the baby's eye.

Don't dig around in the eye with a cloth or a swab. If it stays red, or the baby keeps trying to rub it, or there are a lot of tears in it, go to the doctor.

If there is a chemical in the eye, gently wash the eye with running water for at least ten minutes. Get medical help.

Objects in the ears

Don't try to remove an object stuck in your child's ear, because you could push it farther in.

Sometimes an object has been pushed so far

into the ear that it can't be seen. One sign that this has happened is a very bad-smelling fluid leaking from the ear.

If there is an insect in the ear, drop in a little cooking oil or baby oil. It stops the buzzing and often washes the insect out.

Objects in the nose

Don't try to remove an object stuck in the nose. You may only push it up farther.

Have the child try to blow the object out. If it will not come out this way, get medical help.

Frostbite

Your child has frostbite if the skin is white or greyish, feels very hard and cold, and has no feeling.

Warm the frozen parts against the body or wrap them in extra clothing or cloth. Don't rub with snow or with anything else, and bring the child into a warm place as quickly as possible. Take off any tight clothes.

Soak frozen parts in warm, not hot water, or cover them with warm blankets or towels. Don't use a heating pad or hot-water bottle.

Stop the warming process when the skin becomes pink. As the frostbitten parts begin to warm up, they can become very painful.

Give the child warm drinks.

Get help if the frostbitten areas don't become pink again or if the child has a lot of pain.

Sunburn

Several times a day, apply cloths wrung out in cool water. Calamine lotion might help if the burn is itchy. Keep the child out of the sun for as long as the skin is red.

Get help if the sunburn blisters or swells up. Don't break the blisters.

Prevent sunburn by covering heads with sun hats and by keeping your child out of the sun. Ask your doctor about a sun block cream for your child.

Sunstroke and heat exhaustion

Sunstroke and heat exhaustion are more serious than sunburn. They happen when a child has been out in the sun too long or has been very active in very hot weather.

Cool the child and get medical help.

To prevent sunstroke, give your child more to drink on a hot day. Cover her head with a sunhat and don't let her stay in the sun too long.

Chapter 17

When Your Baby Is Sick

Babies get sick faster than adults, but they also get better faster.

Sometimes you will wonder if your baby is sick. He might be fussy, or in a bad mood, or cry continually. If he doesn't have a fever, is eating well and has regular bowel movements, keep an eye on him and don't worry. He may have a good sleep and wake up back to normal.

Crying
If he is clean and dry, and not hungry or bored, give him a pat and a smile. If he is sick, he will cry again.

A baby in pain will cry loudly and sharply without stopping. If the pain is not acute, he may cry and whine and snuffle.

How can I tell if he is sick?
A sick baby will show one or more of the following symptoms:

- He is very unhappy, irritable or cranky, or very sleepy.
- His crying may be sharp and loud, or weak and whiny.
- He won't eat for several feedings.

- He vomits or throws up more than the usual spitting up after meals.
- He has diarrhea.
- He has a runny nose or a cough; he is hoarse; his breathing is faster than usual or he grunts when he breathes.
- He has a temperature of 37.7°C (100°F) or higher.
- He is very pale or cold.
- He looks flushed with hot, dry skin or is very sweaty.
- He seems droopy and tired, or sleeps more than usual.
- He has a rash.
- He has fits or convulsions.
- His skin keeps peeling.
- He doesn't seem his usual self.

A sick baby will feel better if you hold him and comfort him. Make sure he is in a warm, quiet place. Extra fluids and a lukewarm bath may be all that's necessary to settle the baby and bring his temperature down to normal.

If he has diarrhea, don't give him anything to eat or milk to drink. There are water solutions especially made for babies with diarrhea that you can get at your drugstore. Ask your doctor or nurse about it.

Can my sick child go to day care?

Your child should not go to day care if he is vomiting, or has a fever or diarrhea. Ask a neighbour, family member or friend to help look after him until he is better.

Let your caregiver know about allergies, diet restrictions or other medical conditions that may require prompt attention.

What should I tell the doctor?

When you call the doctor, have the following information ready:

- If the baby has a high temperature, let the doctor know what his temperature has been every two hours.
- If the baby has diarrhea, tell the doctor the times, the colour and whether the movements are loose or have a shape.
- If the baby is throwing up, keep track of how often he throws up, how much, what the vomit looks like, and how the baby looks when he is throwing up.

The more information you can give the doctor, the more help he or she can be.

How to take a baby's temperature

It is hard to take a baby's temperature by mouth, because the baby will not cooperate. Take it in his armpit. Here's how you do it:

1. Shake the thermometer so the reading is 35° C (95° F) or lower.
2. Put it under your baby's arm near the armpit. Hold the arm snugly against the body for five minutes.
3. Take the thermometer out. Don't hold it by the bulb, because that will change the reading. Hold it by the other end. Look for where the

red line stops. The number at the end of the red line is the baby's temperature.

4. Normal temperature taken by armpit should be between 36.0° C and 37.5° C (96.8° F and 99.0° F). A temperature above 40° C (104° F) can be serious.

Another way to tell the baby's temperature is to buy special paper strips at the drugstore.

What should I do when my baby has a fever?

Babies often get higher temperatures than adults, and they peak faster. Try to lower his temperature by dressing him lightly. A T-shirt and diaper are enough; don't wrap him up in blankets. Give him lots of juices or water if he drinks them. Don't give any medicine without checking with your doctor.

Get help if a baby less than six months old has a fever, no matter what the temperature is. Get help for any child who has a fever for longer than forty-eight hours, or if you can't get his temperature to go down to normal (36.0° C to 37.5° C/ 96.8° F to 99.0° F) or if there are other problems as well as the fever—stiff neck, vomiting, diarrhea, earache or rash.

Convulsions

When the baby has a high fever, he occasionally has a convulsion. These look very scary, and it is hard to believe that they are not always as dangerous as they look.

The baby rolls his eyes. He goes stiff and pale.

He waves his arms and legs and passes out. This might last a few minutes.

- Keep calm. Don't try to keep him still, but make sure he can't bump himself on anything hard.
- Don't put anything in his mouth during a convulsion. Children do not swallow their tongues during a convulsion.
- Put him on his side. Keep him in such a position that if he vomits he won't inhale the vomit.
- The baby will drool. Wipe up the saliva around his mouth so he can't inhale it.
- Try to lower his temperature. Give him a warm bath.
- Do not wrap him up. This will just make him hotter.
- Notice how long the convulsion lasts. Notice when it happens. The doctor will want to know.
- If it has not stopped after five minutes, call 911, a doctor or an ambulance, even if you have to leave the child alone to do it.

Call your doctor when your baby has a convulsion so you can find out what caused it. If you can't get your doctor, take the baby to the hospital or clinic.

Stomach aches

Most babies have upset stomachs once in a while. They may refuse their meals, throw up, or have diarrhea or be constipated.

When your baby has an upset stomach, it may be the first sign of illness. Or it may just be that he has been eating too much, or not enough, or not getting enough sleep.

Diarrhea

Diarrhea is something to watch closely. The baby may have an infection, usually caused by germs in his bottle or his formula. The germs could have come from flies or from some other person. Adults or other children in the family may have the same germs, but they may not get diarrhea.

Diarrhea can also be a sign of some other illnesses.

The danger with diarrhea is that the baby could lose too much water. An older child can lose the water without as much danger of dehydration.

Diarrhea often starts with crankiness, then cramps. The diarrhea may be watery and green. It may sound explosive. If it is not taken care of, the baby will lose weight. He may seem weak, and not have much energy.

Call your doctor if:
- there is blood in the diarrhea
- the child has a high fever, 38.5° C (101.3° F) orally or 40° C (104° F) by the armpit method
- the baby is drowsy and refuses to eat or drink
- there are signs of loss of body fluids (dehydration) such as sunken eyes, dry skin or mouth, the baby is urinating less than normal or has dark yellow urine

- there are more than five dirty diapers a day

Your doctor or nurse may suggest you get a fluid replacement from the drugstore; it is made from water with added nutrients.

A breast-fed baby normally has soft or runny bowel movements, but you will know when he has diarrhea because it smells bad.

To protect yourself and the rest of your family, wash your hands very well after you handle the baby or his clothes. It is very important to handle dirty diapers carefully so you don't spread the germs.

If you wash your diapers, make sure they are washed well with hot water and detergent. Rinse them well. Dry them in the sun or in high heat to kill any germs left in them.

If you use disposables, don't leave them lying around. Put them in a garbage bag or garbage can.

How should I feed the baby after he is better?

When the baby's temperature is back to normal, and when the diarrhea seems to be getting better, follow your doctor's instructions. He or she may suggest you give the baby his meals again if he seems to want them.

If the baby was eating solid foods before he got sick, give him solids again. Start with one food at a time, and add them in the same way you did when you first started to give him solids.

Your baby may get mild diarrhea from time to time because of a new food, a change of food, too much food or too much sugar. Stop giving him solid food for a day. If he is on a formula, mix it half and half with boiled water, and give him lots of it. If the stools get firmer the next day, he could have his regular formula, and his regular food the day after.

Throwing up

Babies often spit up after they eat. This is very common. It is not the same as throwing up or vomiting. Spitting up is just getting rid of extra milk. It may show that the baby has been given too much to eat. Maybe he has swallowed air because his bottle was propped up, or maybe the nipple has been letting air in. He will spit up less if you burp him more often. Make sure he doesn't get moved around too much after a meal.

Throwing up or vomiting is something different. If he throws up, stop giving him all solid food.

Get help if:
- the baby spits up after a feeding hard enough to hit the wall or splatter onto the floor
- the vomiting is frequent (three or four times in two hours, for example)
- there is a high fever (38.5° C [101.3° F] orally or 40° C [104° F] by the armpit method) with the vomiting
- your baby is drowsy and refuses to eat or drink
- there are signs of loss of body fluids (dehydration) such as sunken eyes, dry skin or

mouth, the baby is urinating less than normal or has dark yellow urine

It is much more serious if your baby is vomiting and has diarrhea at the same time.

Constipation

The baby is constipated when his stools are hard instead of normally firm. It doesn't matter how often they come; if they are hard, the baby is constipated. Some babies have only one bowel movement every two or three days. Some breast-fed babies have only one stool every five days. This is normal as long as the stools are not hard.

Make sure your baby is getting enough to drink. If he is eating fruit, try giving him a teaspoon or two of strained prunes or apricots every day.

Get help if:
- the problem last more than five days
- there is blood in the stools
- the child cries when he has a bowel movement

If your baby is constipated, it may be a sign that he is not getting enough to eat. If he cries long before he should be hungry, or right after he has eaten, he may not be eating enough. Talk to your doctor. Do not use laxatives or enemas unless your doctor recommends them.

Hiccups

Many babies have hiccups. They will not harm the baby, and they usually don't last very long. Pat the baby on the back, or give him a little more milk or water. If your baby spits up when he hiccups, hold him with his head up.

Colic

Colic is a kind of stomach ache or cramp. Colic attacks can last for as long as three hours and may go on for several weeks. Colic usually disappears by the time the baby is about four months old.

A colicky baby is not ill, but he is in pain. After a feeding, he may cry and pull his knees up to his chest. The baby's abdomen may become firm; he may pass gas. Although rocking, holding, walking, singing and feeding may help for a moment, the baby will start screaming again when he feels the pain.

Colic can occur in both bottle-fed and breast-fed babies. Although it is not known why some babies develop colic, it may be caused by one or more of the following:

- a central nervous system that may not be fully developed
- poor burping methods
- too much or too little food
- swallowing air
- something the baby can't tolerate in his diet, or in his mother's diet if he is being breast-fed

What can I do?

- Give the baby smaller feedings more often.
- Burp the baby before, during and after feedings.
- Don't feed your baby while he is lying down;

hold him so he is sitting partly up.

- Let your baby get a lot of sucking to stimulate his intestinal track. Let him suck on an empty breast or on a soother.
- Check the breast or bottle position to make sure your baby is not swallowing too much air.
- If you are breast-feeding, avoid eating foods that many people are allergic to, such as milk products and citrus fruits.
- Do not get your baby excited. Play soothing or soft music.
- Put your baby on his abdomen or gently massage his abdomen.
- Put a warm cloth on his abdomen or give him a tub bath.
- Rub your baby's back to comfort him and to encourage him to pass gas.
- Use an infant carrier ("snugglie") around the house so that you can still hold and soothe your baby while you do other things.
- Try to avoid extra stress on yourself by getting help with meals and child care, especially in the evening. Try to get extra rest during the afternoon so you will be ready to look after the baby at night.
- Take the baby for a carriage or car ride; the motion and sound often soothes a colicky baby.

Don't get discouraged. Every baby outgrows colic. Yours will too.

Skin troubles

Diaper rash
When your baby has diaper rash, he may just have a few red spots or he may have pimples, blisters and sores. Wet diapers rubbing against the baby's skin give him diaper rash. Although it is very common, blond babies and redheads seem to get it worse than darker babies.

What should I do when my baby has diaper rash?
- Leave the baby's diapers off as much as you can. Air will dry out the rash and promote healing.
- Let the baby sleep without diapers. Put a few diapers on top of the sheet, and lay the baby on his abdomen on top of the diapers.
- Don't use rubber or plastic pants unless you have to.
- Keep the skin under the diaper as dry and clean as you can.
- If you put a diaper on the baby, cover the rash with a thin coat of zinc oxide jelly. Ask your druggist for a good cheap brand.

How can I stop the rash from coming back?
- Change the baby's diapers often.
- Keep the skin under the diaper as clean and dry as you can.
- Don't use rubber or plastic pants unless you have to.

- Look for soap, baby oil, lotions and powders that don't have any perfume in them, because perfume may further irritate diaper rash.
- Rinse the diapers twice. Put half a cup of vinegar in the rinse.
- Try a new kind of diaper. If you use disposable diapers, try cloth ones. If you use cloth, try disposables. See if it makes any difference to your baby's rash.

When should I get help?
Check with a doctor or a public health nurse if:
- there are sores in the rash
- the pimples seem to have pus under them
- the rash is getting worse

Prickly heat
Prickly heat is a rash of tiny blisters that occurs when the weather is hot or when the baby is dressed too warmly. The rash will come out on his face or on the part of his body that has the most clothes covering it.

Take some of his clothes off so he is not too hot. Sponge him off often with a little water. A little baby talcum, baby powder or corn starch might help to keep his skin dry and comfortable.

Eczema
The eczema might be just a red patch or two, or a little scaly patch. There may be red patches that turn into blisters. The blisters will break and the

wetness underneath gets a crust on it. It is very itchy.

Eczema is one of the most common skin rashes. It is found on the cheeks, forehead and head. It may spread to the fronts of the elbows and the backs of the knees. Sometimes the whole body is covered with the rash.

The baby probably gets eczema because he is allergic to something in his food or his home. A baby who has eczema may develop other allergies, such as asthma or hay fever, or the allergies may run in the family.

Eczema may be so itchy that the baby will get very cranky. He will not be able to sleep. He will scratch the red spots and may get them infected.

What should I do if my baby gets eczema?
- Keep the baby's nails cut very short so he can't harm himself too much when he scratches.
- Use cotton clothes. Nylon or wool will make his skin more itchy.
- Use oil to clean the baby's skin. Soap and water will make the eczema worse.

Impetigo
If your child has impetigo, he will have red sores. The sores turn into blisters and the blisters leak, then make scabs that are a yellowish colour. Impetigo sores show up on the face, hands, elbows or knees.

These sores are itchy. Try not to let your child

scratch and pick at them, since the sores can be spread over the body. Impetigo can also be spread if your child touches someone else or if someone else uses your child's towels or sheets.

What should I do?
- Call your doctor. The doctor will probably give your child antibiotics.
- Soak your child's sores in the tub or with clean cloths until the scabs are soft. Wash the sores to help take the scabs off and let the pus come out. **The sores will not get better until the pus is gone.** Soak and wash two or three times a day while you are waiting to see the doctor.
- Wash your hands often. Make sure your child washes his hands often.
- Cut your child's nails.
- Don't let anyone else use your child's sheets or towels. Keep them away from the rest of the family's towels and sheets. Wash them often.

Thrush

Thrush is caused by a fungus growing in the lining of the mouth. If your baby has thrush, you will see white spots on the inside of the cheeks, gums and tongue. It is easy to confuse thrush with white milk curds in the baby's mouth. However, milk curds wipe off very easily and don't leave a mark behind.

Thrush doesn't bother most babies, and

usually it clears up with no trouble. Your doctor will give you some medicine if it is needed.

Colds

Try to keep your baby from getting a cold. If you have a cold, always wash your hands before and after you handle him. Try to limit his contact with visitors who have colds.

Babies with colds usually lose their appetites.

What should I do if my baby has a cold?

- Keep his room draft-free and warm (22° C or 72° F).
- Don't let him get cold. Don't give him a bath if the room is not warm enough.
- Use a cool-mist humidifier to put some humidity into the room. Put it in a safe place.
- Give him extra water to drink. Give him his usual meals if he wants them.
- Keep cigarette smoke away from your baby.
- Don't use any nose drops or cough or cold medicine unless your doctor tells you to. Most colds go away without medicines, and some medicines have side effects for babies.

When should I get help?

Call your doctor if:

- the baby cries and moves his head from side to side (he may have an earache)
- the baby has trouble breathing, or breathes very quickly and has a cough
- the baby doesn't get better after a few days

- the baby has an earache with the cold
- the baby has a temperature of over 38.5° C (101.3° F) orally or 40°C (104°F) by the armpit method
- the baby has a stiff neck
- the baby has a bad cough, chest pain and high fever

Sore throat

It is often hard to tell when a baby has a sore throat. If he has trouble swallowing, he may have a sore throat, especially if he is also fussy, flushed or feverish and does not want to eat. Most sore throats are uncomfortable but not harmful. However, strep throat can lead to other, more serious illnesses.

Keep the child quiet and comfortable, and give lots of fluids like water, juice and popsicles.

When should I get help?

If your child has a fever with the sore throat, check with a doctor. If the doctor gives you a prescription, be sure your child takes the medication until it is finished. Your child may seem to feel better very quickly, but the germs that caused the illness will not be gone until all the medicine has been taken.

Croup

Children with croup make a dry, barking noise when they inhale. They have trouble breathing. Sometimes a cold or a runny nose turns into

232

croup; sometimes croup comes on suddenly (usually at night) with no other symptoms.

Although it is very scary, don't panic.

If your child is having trouble breathing, there are two things you can do:

1. Wrap him up warmly and go out into the cold damp air; OR
2. Take him into the bathroom, close the door and turn on a cold shower. Let him breathe the damp air as the shower runs.

When should I get help?
Get help if:
- your child has a high fever
- your child is drooling
- breathing has not improved after ten minutes

Earache
Since your baby can't talk to you about a sore ear, it is sometimes hard to tell if he has an earache. Young children sometimes pull or rub at the sore ear or at the side of the head.

Earaches are serious. If they are not taken care of, the baby's hearing may be damaged.

Don't put anything in your child's ear before checking with the doctor.

When should I get help?
Any earache should be checked by a doctor. If the child has a fever with the earache, or has pus leaking from the ear, call a doctor immediately.

Parasites

Lice

Lice are tiny black bugs that live in hair. They lay eggs, called nits, which look like little white pieces of dandruff and stick to the hair. Lice are very common. They are very itchy, and they spread easily. Anyone can catch lice. It has nothing to do with being dirty.

Drugstores sell a special shampoo or lotion for treating lice. Follow the directions because you need to be careful with it.

When should I get help?

Check with a doctor before treating a baby, or if you are pregnant or breast-feeding.

For children five and under, check with a doctor or public health nurse if the lice don't go away after the first treatment.

If you need advice, call your public health nurse or your doctor.

Scabies

Scabies is an itchy red rash caused when the scabies mite burrows under the skin and lays eggs there. Scabies usually shows up between the fingers, on the wrist or forearms and on the inside of the thighs. The rash starts as tiny bites or blisters, then becomes red and swollen. It always seems itchiest at night.

Drugstores sell a special cream or lotion for treating scabies, but you need to be careful with it. Follow the directions on the container.

When should I get help?

Check with a doctor before treating a baby, or if you are pregnant or breast-feeding.

Check with a doctor or public health nurse if the scabies doesn't go away after the first treatment.

If you need advice, call your public health nurse or your doctor.

Pinworms

Pinworms live in the intestines. They are usually discovered when someone notices that the child is scratching around the rectum, especially at night. The worms are small and thin and white. Sometimes you can see them if you look at the child's rectum after he has been asleep for about an hour.

See your doctor for a prescription for some medicine.

Be prepared to treat the whole family. Pinworms are so contagious that if one person has them, everyone probably has them.

Trim and scrub everyone's fingernails.

Make sure the whole family washes their hands after using the toilet and before eating.

Wash everyone's pyjamas, sheets and towels. Wash stuffed animals and toys that your children play with.

Keep your child away from other children until the worms have been treated.

Emergency Delivery

Once in a while the mother can't get to the hospital to have her baby. This part of the book is for you if you have to deliver the baby without help. Try to get help from a doctor or a nurse. While you are looking after the mother, someone else should keep phoning the hospital or the doctor. Sometimes you can get help over the phone, even if you can't get to the hospital.

Keep the mother and baby clean

If you keep things clean, you can help protect the mother from getting an infection. Wash your hands with soap and water before you start. Put on a clean apron.

You will need:

- clean towels to put under the mother
- newspapers to keep the bed clean
- two or three clean cloths, handkerchiefs or pieces of gauze
- a clean blanket or a big bath towel to wrap the baby in
- six sanitary pads
- big bags to hold all the garbage
- a wash basin or bowl
- a clean apron for you to wear

Labour and Delivery

Labour has three parts. If you know about the three parts, you can make a good guess about how much time you have left before the baby is born.

Usually the first part lasts many hours. If this is a first baby, the first part of labour may last more than twelve hours. It will be less than that if it is a second or third child.

During this first part, the lower end of the uterus slowly opens up. It opens far enough to let the baby's head through.

Sometimes all the stages are much faster, and you may need to make an emergency delivery.

Labour pains are mild at first. They come about twenty minutes apart. As labour moves along, the pains get very regular and start to come as close together as two or three minutes.

Try to let the mother know everything will be okay. Try to help her relax and rest between pains. She shouldn't try to push. Don't tell her to push until she feels the need to push. This will be in the second part of labour. In the first part, she should just relax.

The second part is much shorter than the first part. The lower end of the uterus is completely open and the baby can be pushed out. The mother wants to push with every pain. Pains are now less than five minutes apart. The mother takes a deep breath and holds it. Then she pushes or bears down.

You will be able to see the baby's hair and

head. It might look a bit grey and purple. After the head comes out, feel at the back of the baby's neck. If there is a loop of the cord around the baby's neck, gently loosen it and slip it over the head.

Wipe the baby's mouth, nose and eyes with a clean soft cloth. Don't use anything made of paper. The head will turn to one side or the other. This will let the shoulders come out.

You can help the shoulders come out. The shoulder that is highest can come out first. Hold the baby's head and neck. Let them drop down a little, and the shoulder will come out. Then lift the head a little, and the other shoulder will come out. The rest of the baby will come out quickly after the shoulders are born.

Try to hold the baby as he is being born. Hold him so his head and shoulders are lower than the rest of the body. This will let the liquid drain out of his mouth and nose. You will need both hands to hold the baby because he will be slippery and wet.

Taking care of the baby

Place the baby across the mother's tummy and cover them both with towels or blankets. Be careful not to pull on the cord. The cord is still attached to the mother.

If the baby doesn't start to cry right away, hold him with his head lower than his bum and massage firmly along the back from the bum up to the shoulders. If the baby still doesn't breathe, you will have to give him little puffs of air from your mouth. Tilt the baby's head back just a little; cover his nose and mouth with your mouth, and gently blow. Puff in just the air you have in your cheeks. Don't blow too hard. You should see the baby's chest lift up a tiny bit.

Getting the baby to breathe and keeping him warm are the important things. The room should at least 23° C (74° F).

Take the mother and the baby to the hospital as soon as possible. You may wish to call an ambulance to do this.

After the baby is born

The only thing left after the baby is born is for the placenta to be born. The placenta is a round, dark red organ that fed the baby before he was born. It comes out in the third stage of labour. It usually comes out about twenty or thirty minutes after the baby is born.

To check on the progress of the placenta, press gently on the mother's stomach. You will feel the uterus get hard. It is pushing out the placenta. You will see the cord getting longer and longer. Do not pull on it. Just let it come out. Finally the placenta will come out in a gush of blood.

When the placenta is born, wrap it and the cord in with the baby. Make sure the baby has a clear space to breathe. It will be messy, but the baby will be fine. The baby will not lose any blood. The baby's blood does not move through the placenta after he is born.

You can leave the baby on the mother's stomach for twenty minutes or so. The baby pressing down helps the uterus to go back to its old size and helps stop bleeding. The mother will be happy to see the baby and touch him. It is dangerous to the baby if you tie and cut the cord, because it is hard to keep things clean enough. The baby might get an infection. Wait for medical help to do this.

Looking after the mother

There is only one thing left to look out for. Sometimes the muscles of the uterus do not tighten up to make the uterus go back to normal. The mother will start to bleed too much. You can rub her tummy just near her bellybutton, or she can do it herself. This helps the uterus tighten.

Don't let the mother sit up. Watch her closely for at least an hour. Keep her lying down with her head low. Put some newspaper covered with a clean towel under her hips. Put a sanitary pad in place.

She may feel better if you wipe her hands and face with warm water. She should have a sweet drink.

Check the pad every once in a while. Watch for too much bleeding. Here are some signs of too much bleeding: she is restless; her skin is damp and cool; or her pulse rate is high. If you see any of these signs, get medical help immediately. Don't move the mother yourself.

If an hour goes by with no trouble, the mother

will probably be okay. You can move her and the baby to the hospital. Here the doctor or nurse or midwife will clamp and cut the cord. This will be done with clamps and sterile scissors.

If you can't get the mother and baby to the hospital right away, it is not a great emergency. The baby will be okay for several hours just as he is.

Emergencies that sometimes happen

The baby is already born when you get there
Sometimes the baby is already born when you get there. You may find the baby lying between the mother's legs. There might be a pool of liquid that the baby is lying in. Lift the baby gently by the feet, holding the head with your other hand. Hold the baby with his head down so that the fluid can drain out of his nose and mouth. This will make it easier for him to breathe. Wipe his mouth and eyes. Wrap him in a warm towel or blanket and put him across his mother's tummy. Now you are ready to wait for the placenta to be born. Look back at the section called "After the baby is born" for help with the placenta.

The baby is born bottom first
Nearly always the baby is born head first. Sometimes he is born bottom first. This is called a breech birth.

Again, your job is to wait for the baby to be born. Let him come on his own. Do not pull on the body or on the legs or arms.

Wrap a warm towel around the body as it comes out. This will keep the baby warm. If he is cold, he may take a gasp of air. You don't want the baby to gasp for air because his head has not been born yet, and there is no air for him to breathe inside his mother.

The baby's weight will gradually bring him out. Then you can help. Wait until the shoulders and arms have come out and you can see the back of his neck and some of the hair on his head. Then hold his feet between the thumb and fingers of one hand. Lift the legs and body up in a half circle. When you lift his legs you will see his nose and mouth come out. Gently wipe the nose and mouth, and any fluid in the airway can run out. The baby will be able to breathe. Don't pull. Ask the mother to take short panting breaths. The rest of the head should come out in a few minutes.

If you can do this slowly and carefully, you will help the mother and baby a lot. Wrap the baby up warmly. Put him across his mother's tummy. Now you can wait for the placenta to be born. Look back at the section called "After the baby is born" for help with the placenta.

The baby is born on the way to the hospital

If you are on the way to the hospital, and you know that the baby will be born before you get there, don't go through red lights. Stop the car so the baby can be born.

Your job is to help keep the mother calm and to wait for the baby. The baby will be born; you

242

just have to catch it. Keep the baby warm by wrapping him in a coat or blanket or whatever is available. Make sure the baby breathes. Rub the baby's back if he doesn't breathe on his own.

Get someone to drive you, the mother and the baby to the hospital once the baby is born.

Index

A

Abdomen exercises
  after delivery, 111-113
  during pregnancy, 62
Accident prevention,
  184-187
Additives to food, 46
Advice (on baby care), 102
Aerobics, during pregnancy,
  51
Affection, showing to baby,
  98, 100, 172
Afterbirth (placenta), 17, 19,
  83, 239-240
Afterpains, 91, 92, 130
AIDS and pregnancy, 10
Airplane travel
  during pregnancy, 52-53
  with baby, 163-164
Alcohol, drinking during
  pregnancy, 7, 8, 19, 47
Allergies, of baby
  and breast-feeding, 127
  and eczema, 228-229
  insect stings, 212
Amniocentesis, 35
Amniotic fluid, 77-78
Amniotic sac, 17, 87
Anemia, of baby, 34
Anesthetic during labour, 85
Anger, 174-175
Appearance, of newborn, 84
Appetite, of baby
  normal, 150-151
  in sickness, 216, 231
Appetite, during pregnancy,
  44-45

B

Baby seats, 190
Baby sitters, 177-178
Back injuries, 210
Backache and labour, 77
Basements, accident
  prevention, 194-195
Basic baby supplies, 67-75
Bathrooms, accident
  prevention, 192-193
Bath, of baby
  preparation, 119-121
  sponge, 121-122
  tub, 123-124
Bath, of mother
  after delivery, 92
  during pregnancy, 53
Bed, of baby, 68-69, 190
Bellybutton, of baby, 119
Birth
  emergency procedures,
    236-243
  preparation in prenatal
    classes, 36- 37
  stages, 81-83
Birth control
  after delivery, 93, 99
  methods, 103-108
  before pregnancy, 8-9
Birth defects, 9, 97
Birthmarks, 116
Bites, 212

Bleeding, baby, 211-212
Bleeding, mother
  during emergency
  delivery, 240
  before labour, 77
  during pregnancy, 30
Boating safety, 197
Blood, Rh factor, 8, 33-34.
  See also Bleeding
Body, of baby
  bathing, 122
  after birth, 84
Body, of mother
  after delivery, 92-93
  during pregnancy, 24-30
Bonding, with baby, 83, 85,
  98, 100, 127
Bones, broken, 198, 209-210
Bottles, nursing
  bedtime, 141, 159
  how to give, 139-141
  preparing formula, 137-139
  sterilizing, 137, 138
  supplies, 73
Bowel movements, of baby
  constipated, 224
  diarrhea, 221-222
  normal, 116, 132
Bras, during pregnancy, 54
Braxton-Hicks
  contractions, 76
Breast-feeding
  and birth control, 93
  and colic, 226
  after delivery, 91
  and eating well, 39
  milk, expressed, 132, 133,
    134, 135
  milk, frozen, 133-134
  partner's role, 126
  and uterus, 127, 130

weaning, 135-136
and working, 132-133
Breasts, of baby, 116
Breasts, during pregnancy,
  24
Breathing, baby
  during emergency
  delivery, 238-239
  rescue, 205-207
  during sickness, 217
Breathing, mother
  during labour, 78-79
  and relaxation, 63-64
Breech birth, 241-242
Burns, 198, 199-200
Burping, 141

C
Caesarean birth, 86-87, 130
Calcium, 41-42, 46
Canada's Food Guide, 44,
  45
Car seat, baby, 73, 163,
  187-189
Carbohydrates, 41
Carbon monoxide (in
  cigarette smoke), 52
Care of baby. *See* specific
  topics, such as Bath,
  Feeding, Holding, etc.
Care of mother. *See* specific
  topics, such as Labour,
  Pregnancy, Rest, etc.
Caregivers, 177-180
Cat litter, 56
Catheter, 86
Cavities, 141, 159-160
Cereals, 144
Cervical cap, 107
Cervix,
  and I.U.D., 105

before labour, 77, 78
and reproduction, 14
Checkups
after delivery, 99
before pregnancy, 8-9
during pregnancy, 24-26, 31
Chemicals
accident prevention, 192, 193, 194, 197
avoidance during pregnancy, 56
emergency procedures, 200
Chewing, 161
Child care, 51, 177-183
Childbirth education classes, 36-37
Children, older, 67, 75, 100, 126, 177
Chlamydia, 10
Choking, 140, 198, 200-205
Cigarette smoking, and pregnancy, 7, 8, 19, 52
Circumcision, 35-36, 118
Classes, childbirth education, 36-37
Clothes, of baby, 69-70, 125, 154
Clothes, during pregnancy, 54
Coaching, during labour, 38, 75, 88-89
Cocaine, 55
Colds, 231-232
Colic, 225-226
Commercial baby food, 147
Community services, 1, 32, 37, 91, 136
Conception
and breast-feeding, 93
description, 16
Condoms, 106, 107-108

Confidence
of baby, 172
of mother, 37, 95-96
See also Trust
Consistency of solid foods, 145-146
Constipation, of baby, 224
Constipation, during pregnancy, 28, 45
Contraception
after delivery, 93, 99
methods, 103-108
before pregnancy, 8-9
Contractions, during labour, 76, 77, 79, 81, 82, 83
Contracts, day-care, 181
Convulsions, 217, 219-220
Cord, umbilical. See Umbilical cord
Coughs, of baby, 232
Cradle cap, 122
Cramps, of mother
leg, during pregnancy, 28
uterine, 77, 91, 92, 130
Cream, spermicidal, 106, 107
Crib, 68-69, 190
Crying, of baby, 117-118, 216-217
Crying, of mother, 26-27, 94, 101-102
C-section, 86-87, 130
Cuts, 211
Cutting nails, 124

D
Danger
foods for baby, 146
household accidents, 184-186

symptoms during
  pregnancy, 30-31
Day care
  considerations, 178-182
  during sickness, 217-218
Defects, birth, 9, 97
Dehydration, 221, 223-224
Delivery
  due date, 17, 18
  emergency procedures,
    236-243
  preparation in childbirth
    education classes, 36-37
  stages of labour, 80-83
Dental care
  of baby, 159-161
  during pregnancy, 9, 26
Depression, 26-27, 94,
  101-102
Development of baby,
  165-172
Diabetes and labour, 87
Diaper rash, 71, 227-228
Diaper service, 72
Diapers, 70-72, 73, 125
Diaphragm, 105, 106
Diarrhea, of baby, 217, 218,
  220, 221-222, 224
Diet. *See* Eating, Feeding,
  Food, Nutrition
Dieting, and pregnancy, 44
Diphtheria, 161, 162
Discharge, vaginal
  during breast-feeding, 130
  after delivery, 93, 130
  at onset of labour, 77
  during pregnancy, 53, 54
Discipline, 173-174
Doctor, importance of
    seeing
  after accidents, 198-215

for emergency delivery, 236
  during pregnancy, 24-31
  for sick child, 216-235
Douching during
  pregnancy, 54
Drinking (alcohol) during
  pregnancy, 7, 8, 19, 47
Driveways, accident
  prevention, 196
Drooling, 161
Drowsiness, of baby, 210,
  216, 217
Drugs
  effect on baby, 7, 19
  and sexually transmitted
    diseases, 10
  use of medication during
    pregnancy, 54-55
Due date (delivery), 17, 18

E
Ears, of baby
  on airplanes, 163
  earaches, 231, 232, 233
  infections, 141
  objects in, 213-214
  protrusion of (sticking
    out), 115
  washing, 121-122
Eating, baby
  by herself/himself, 169,
    170, 171
  mealtimes, 150-151
  and sickness, 216-217,
    222-224
  See also Feeding, Food,
    Nutrition
Eating, during pregnancy,
  39-47
Eczema, 228-229
Electrical appliances,

accident prevention, 192, 193, 195
Embryo, growth of, 17, 21
Emergency
  delivery, 236-243
  telephone numbers, 178, 186
Emotions. *See* Crying, Depression, Feelings, Laughter, Smiling
Epidural anesthetic, 85, 86
Episiotomy, 83, 85
Exercise, of baby, 157
Exercise, of mother
  after Caesarean birth, 87
  after delivery, 92, 109- 113
  during pregnancy, 7, 51, 58-62
Expressed milk, 132, 133, 134, 135
Eyes, of baby
  after birth, 84
  colour, 115
  focussing, 115
  injuries, 213
  washing, 121

F
Face, of baby
  after birth, 115
  washing, 121
Fallopian tubes, 13-14, 108
Falls, accidental, 209-210
Family
  allowance, 99
  closeness, 99-100, 117, 177
  health history, 8, 9
  planning, 103-108
Farm safety, 197
Fathers
  bonding with baby, 100
  decisions during

  pregnancy, 56-57
  eating during pregnancy, 47
  feelings, 75
  holding baby, 125
  as labour coach, 38, 75, 88-89
  lifestyle changes caused by baby, 10-11
  and parenting, 164, 182
  preparation for childbirth, 37-38
  and relaxation exercises, 66
  sharing responsibility for baby, 1, 2, 126, 182-183
Fears, of baby, 169, 170, 176
Feeding
  bottle, 127-128, 136-141
  breast, 127, 128-136
  commercial baby food, 147
  cow's milk, 143
  dangerous foods, 146
  drinking from cup, 141-142
  formula, 136-139
  homemade food, 147-148
  mealtimes, 150- 151
  partner's role, 126
  solid foods, 143-148
  vegetarian diet, 148- 149
  vitamins and minerals, 149
  water, 142-143
  See also Eating, Food, Nutrition
Feelings
  after delivery, 83, 86-87, 90, 93-96, 100, 101-102
  during pregnancy, 26-27, 55-56
Fertility, 106-107
Fertilization (of egg), 15-16
Fetus, development of, 17, 21-22

Fever, baby, 219
Fever, during pregnancy, 31
Fibre, 41, 42
Fingernails, cutting, 124
Fire prevention, 192, 193, 194, 195
First aid
  procedures, 199-215
  supplies, 186-187
Fish, 42-43
Fluoride, 149-150
Foam, spermicidal, 105, 106, 107
Folic acid, 41, 42, 46
Food
  additives, 46
  costs, 46-47
  groups, 40-43
  See also Eating, Feeding, Nutrition
Forceps, 86
Forms, filling out, 99
Formula, infant
  kinds of, 136-137
  preparing, 137-139
Fractures, 209-210
Frostbite, 214
Fruit, 41-42, 145, 146, 149

G
General anesthetic, 85, 86
Genetic tests, 9
German measles
  immunization against, 92, 162
  and pregnancy, 8, 10, 25
Gonorrhea, 10
Grandparents, 177
Grasp reflex, 167
Growth
  of embryo, 17, 19
  of fetus, 21-22
  during first year, 152-153, 165-171
Guns, accident prevention, 196

H
Hair
  of newborn, 84
  washing, 122
Halls, accident prevention, 194
Head, of baby
  after birth, 84
  injuries to, 198, 210
  during labour, 78, 80, 81, 82, 83
  lifting, 167
  need for support, 115
Headaches, mother, 31
Health, and pregnancy, 2, 47
Hearing, of baby, 171
Heart disease, and labour, 87
Heartburn, during pregnancy, 27-28, 32, 45
Heat exhaustion, 215
Hemoglobin tests, 8
Hemorrhoids, during pregnancy, 29-30
Heroin, 55
Herpes, 10
Hiccups, 224-225
Highchairs, 169, 191
Holding the baby
  in baths, 120, 121, 122, 123
  during bottle-feeding, 139-141
  during breast-feeding, 128, 130
  and burping, 141

and trust, 114, 117
Homemade baby food,
  147-148
Hormones, 94, 95, 102
Hospital
  admission, 78
  filling out forms, 99
  and instruction in baby
    care, 96, 97
  length of stay, 91-92
  preparing for, 73-74
Hot tubs, during pregnancy,
  54
Household cleaners, during
  pregnancy, 56

I

I.U.D. (intrauterine device),
  104-105
Immunization, of mother,
  9-10, 92
Immunization, of baby,
  161-163
Impetigo, 229-230
Incision, after Caesarean
  birth, 87, 92
Incubators, 98
Induced labour, 87-88
Infections, of baby
  colds and sore throats,
    231-233
  diarrhea, 221- 222
  ears, 141, 213-214, 233
  rashes and sores, 227-230
  umbilical cord, 118
Infections, of mother
  after delivery, 93
  during pregnancy, 54
Insecticides, during
  pregnancy, 56
Intercourse, and pregnancy,

15-16
Intrauterine device (I.U.D.),
  104-105
Intravenous tube, 86
Introducing new foods,
  146-147
Ipecac syrup, 200
Iron, 41, 42, 43, 46, 143, 144,
  149
Isolettes, 98
Itchiness, of baby, 227, 228,
  229, 230, 234, 235
Itchiness, after delivery, 92

J

Jaundice, 34, 116
Jelly, spermicidal, 105, 106,
  107
Juices, fruit, 42, 145

K

Kicking in uterus, 21, 30
Kitchens, accident
  prevention, 192

L

Labour
  emergency delivery,
    237-238
  induced, 87-88
  pain relief, 84- 85
  positions, 80, 81
  and relaxation, 62
  signs of, 76-78
  stages, 78, 80-83
Language development, 170
Laughter, during
  pregnancy, 55, 57
Learning, baby
  exploring, 172
  talking, 169, 170

Leaving baby alone,
  avoidance of, 120,
    184-185, 189, 192, 195,
    197
Legs, of baby, 115
Legs, during pregnancy,
  28-29
Lice, 234
Life jackets, 197
Lifting, during pregnancy,
  50, 52
"Lightening," 76
Local anesthetic, 85
Lochia, 93
Lockjaw (tetanus), 161, 162
Lying positions, during
  pregnancy, 64-65

M

Massage, during labour, 80
Maternity
  benefits, 50-51
  clothes, 54
  See also Pregnancy
Mattress, of baby, 68, 190
Measles
  German, 8, 10, 25, 92, 162
  red, 162
Meat, 42-43, 145, 146
Medication during
  pregnancy, 54-55
Menstruation
  after delivery, 93
  during pregnancy, 24
Microwave ovens
  and baby bottles, 139
  and frozen breast milk,
    134
Milk, cow's, 40-41, 46, 143
Minerals, 41, 42, 149
Moods

after delivery, 93-96
  during pregnancy, 26-27
Morning sickness, 27
Moro reflex, 167
Mother, care of
  after delivery, 91-92, 126
  during pregnancy, 24-31,
    37-38, 56-57
Mouth, of baby
  during breast-feeding,
    128-129
  dental care, 159-161
Mouth-to-mouth
  resuscitation
  of baby, 205-206
  of child, 206-209
Movement in womb, 21, 30
Multiple births, 16, 97, 135
Mucous plug, 77
Mumps, 162

N

Nannies, 179, 180
Naps, baby, 155
Nausea. *See* Morning
  sickness, Vomiting
Natural birth control,
  106-107
Neck injuries, 210
Newborn, appearance of, 84
Nicotine and fetus, 7, 8, 19,
  52
Nipples, of baby, 116
Nipples, of mother, 128-130
Nose, of baby
  cleaning, 121
  objects in, 214
Nurse, public health, 152
Nursing, how to, 128-130
Nutrition
  of baby, 127-151

of mother, during
    pregnancy, 39-47
    See also Eating, Feeding,
    Food

O

Older children, and new
    baby, 67, 75, 100, 126, 177
Older mothers, 33
Outdoor clothing, 154
Ovaries, 13, 14
Ovulation, 15
Ovum, 13-15

P

Pacifiers. *See* Soothers
Pain, of baby
    and crying, 216
    colic, 225-226
Pain, of mother
    after delivery, 91, 92, 130
    during labour, 79-80, 84-85
Pap smear, 8
Parasites, 234-235
Parental leave, 50-51
Parenting, 5-6
Partners
    bonding with baby, 100
    decisions during
        pregnancy, 56-57
    eating during pregnancy, 47
    feelings, 75
    holding baby, 126
    as labour coach, 38, 75,
        88-89
    lifestyle changes caused by
        baby, 10-11
    and parenting, 164, 182
    preparation for childbirth,
        37-38
    and relaxation exercises, 66

sharing responsibility for
    baby, 1, 2, 126, 182-183
Pelvis
    and reproduction, 14
    exercises, 61-62, 109-111
Penis, and reproduction, 14,
    15
Penis, of baby, 122
Period, menstrual
    after delivery, 93
    during pregnancy, 24
Personality of baby, 114
Pertussis (whooping cough),
    161, 162
Pets, and babies, 195
Piles (hemorrhoids), during
    pregnancy, 29-30
Pillows
    in baby's crib, 68
    during pregnancy, 64, 65
Pinworms, 235
Placenta
    after delivery, 83
    emergency delivery,
        239-240
    and reproduction, 17, 19
Plants, poisonous, 193
Plastic pants, 227
Playing, 155, 156, 170,
    172-173, 175-176
Playpens, 156, 190
Poisons and chemicals
    accident prevention, 192,
        193, 194, 197
    avoidance during
        pregnancy, 56
    emergency procedures, 200
Polio, 162
Posture, during pregnancy,
    58-60
Poultry, 42-43

Pregnancy
  danger signs, 30-31
  feelings during, 26-27,
    55-56
  length of, 17, 18
  nutrition, 39-47
  and physical health, 7-10
  superstitions, 31-32
  symptoms, 24, 27-30
  tests, 24
Premature babies, 97, 135
Prenatal classes, 36-37
Preparing for baby, 67-75
Preservatives in food, 46
Prickly heat, 228
Protein
  baby's diet, 145
  mother's diet, 41, 43
Public health nurse, 152
Pudendal block, 85
Pushing, during labour,
  81-83

R
Rashes, 234-235
Rectum, of baby, 122
Reflexes, of baby, 167-168
Registration, birth, 99
Relationship, with baby. *See*
  Affection, Bonding, Older
  Children, Relatives
Relatives, 177
Relaxation
  during labour, 78-80
  during pregnancy, 48,
    62-64
Reproductive organs
  female, 13-14
  male, 14-15
Rest
  after delivery, 100

  during hospital stay, 91
  during pregnancy, 48, 50
Resuscitation,
    mouth-to-mouth
  of baby, 205-206
  of child, 206-209
Rh factor, 8, 33-34
Rhythm method (of birth
  control), 106-107
Rooting reflex, 167-168
Routine, of baby, 155
Rubbers (condoms),
  107-108
Rubella (German measles)
  immunization against, 92,
    162
  and pregnancy, 8, 10, 25

S
Safes (condoms), 107-108
Safety
  avoiding accidents and
    injuries, 184-199
  while bathing baby, 120, 121
  in the car, 188-189
  and discipline, 173
  in the home, 192-196
  outdoors, 196-198
  toys, 157
  water, 196, 197
Safety pins, 71, 72
Sanitary napkins, 93
Saunas during pregnancy,
  54
Scabies, 234-235
Scrotum
  adult, 14
  of baby, 116, 122
Semen, and reproduction,
  15
Sex, during pregnancy, 53

Sex, of baby
  and amniocentesis, 35
  superstitions, 32
Sexually transmitted
  diseases, 8, 10
Shoes, during pregnancy, 54
Showers, of mother
  after delivery, 92
  during pregnancy, 53
Sickness, symptoms,
  216-217
Single parents, 5
Sitters, 177-178
Sitting up, 169, 170
Skin, during pregnancy, 29
Skin, of baby
  bathing, 119-124
  at birth, 116
  problems, 227-230, 234-235
Sleep, during pregnancy, 27,
  48
Sleep, of baby, 117, 120,
  154-156
Slivers, 213
Smiles, of baby, 167, 168
Smoking, during pregnancy,
  7, 8, 19, 52
Snack foods, 41, 43-44
Snowmobile safety, 197-198
Soap, 120
Social activities, 51, 102, 183
Soft spot (on baby's head),
  115
Solid foods, 144-148
Soothers, 157-158, 163
Sores, 229-231
Sounds, and baby, 167, 169,
  170, 171
Spanking, avoidance of, 173
Special needs babies, 97,
  100-101

Speech development, 170
Sperm
  and birth control, 105-108
  and reproduction, 15
Spermicides, 105-107
Spitting up, 141, 223
Splints, 209-210
Sponge bath, 121-122
Sponge, vaginal, 106
Sports, during pregnancy,
  51
Sprains, 209-210
Stages of labour, 78, 79,
  80-83
Stairs, accident prevention,
  194
Standing, of baby, 169, 170,
  171
Standing, during pregnancy,
  50
Startle reflex, 167
STDs (sexually transmitted
  diseases), 8
Sterilization (birth control),
  108
Sterilizing bottles, 137-138
Stings, insect, 212-213
Stitches, after delivery, 83,
  91, 92
Stockings, during
  pregnancy, 54
Stomach, of mother
  exercises, 62, 111-113
  pain, during pregnancy, 31
  upset, 45
Stomach aches, baby,
  colic, 225-226
  from formula, 137
  upset, 220-221
Stool, of baby. See Bowel
  movements

Storage rooms, accident prevention, 194-195
Stoves, accident prevention, 192
Strangers, fear of, 169, 170
Strep throat, 232
Stress, during pregnancy, 55-56
Stretch marks, 29
Subsidies, day-care, 181-182
Sucking
  during breast-feeding, 128-130
  thumb, 158-159
Suction, during birth, 86
Sunburn, 215
Sunstroke, 215
Superstitions, about pregnancy, 31-32
Supplies, basic
  bath, 72-73
  bottles, 73
  car seat, 73
  clothes, 69- 70
  crib, 68-69, 190
  diapers, 70-72
Swallowing, 129
Swelling, ankles or feet during pregnancy, 30
Syphilis, 10

T
Talking, by baby, 169, 170
Teenage mothers, 32-33
Teeth, of baby
  avoidance of sweets, 158
  caring for, 159-161
  and fluoride, 149-150
  teething, 160-161
  and thumb-sucking, 158-159
  and Vitamin C during pregnancy, 42
Temperature, of baby
  and clothing, 154
  and crying, 118
  and illness, 217, 218-219
  taking, 218-219
TENS (Transcutaneous Electrical Nerve Stimulation), 80
Testicles, and reproduction, 14
Tetanus (lockjaw), 161, 162, 211, 212
Thirst, during pregnancy, 45
Throat problems, 230-233
Throwing up. *See* Vomiting
Thrush, 230-231
Thumb-sucking, 158-59
Time out, 174
Tiredness, of mother
  after delivery, 94, 95
  before pregnancy, 7
  during pregnancy, 27, 48
Toenails, cutting, 124
Tooth decay, of baby. *See* Cavities
Toxoplasmosis, 56
Toys, 156, 157
Transcutaneous Electrical Nerve Stimulation (TENS), 80
Transition stage of labour, 80
Travel
  with baby, 163-164
  during pregnancy, 52-53
Trust, development of, 114, 117, 156
Tub bath, 123-124
Tubal ligation, 108
Twins, 16, 135

U

U.I. (unemployment
  insurance), 50
Ultrasound, 35
Umbilical cord
  during bath, 122
  caring for, 118-119
  clamping, 84
  during emergency
    delivery, 240, 241
  and placenta, 19
Unconscious baby, 200,
  207-209, 210
Urination
  frequency before birth, 76
  during labour, 80
  during pregnancy, 24, 61
Uterus
  contractions during
    breast-feeding, 91, 127, 130
  after delivery, 92
  and I.U.D., 104
  and placenta, 17
  and reproduction, 13
  shrinking after birth, 92

V

Vaccination, baby, 161-162
Vagina, of baby, 116, 122
Vagina, of mother
  and birth control, 105, 106
  after delivery, 92, 93
  discharge during
    breast-feeding, 130
  discharge during
    pregnancy, 30
  and I.U.D., 105
  before labour, 76-77
  and reproduction, 14
Varicose veins, 28-29, 50, 54
Vasectomy, 108

Vegetables, 41-42, 145, 149
Vegetarian diet, 43, 47,
  148-149
Venereal diseases, 8, 10
Vernix, 84
Visualization, during
  labour, 79-80
Vitamins, 41, 42, 43, 45-46,
  143, 149
Vomiting, by baby, 200,
  210, 217, 218, 223-224
Vomiting, by mother, 24,
  27, 31

W

Walking, by baby, 171, 191
Walking, during pregnancy,
  51
Washing baby. See Bath
Water
  breaking, at onset of
    labour, 77-78
  drinking of, by baby,
    142- 143
  fluoridation, 149-150
  safety, 196-197
Water beds, 68, 194
Weaning, 135-136
Weight, of baby, 131,
  152-153
Weight, of mother, during
  pregnancy, 31, 44
Whooping cough
  (pertussis), 161, 162
Withdrawal (birth control),
  108
Womb. See Uterus
Working
  and breast-feeding, 132-133
  and day care, 178-182
  during pregnancy, 48-50

Worms
  from pets, 195
  pinworms, 235

X
X-rays, during pregnancy,
  26